# Somatic Art Therapy

This book focuses on somatic art therapy for treating acute or chronic pain, especially resulting from physical and/or psychological trauma. It discusses the role of the psyche in physical healing and encourages combining of traditional medicine and holistic perspectives in treatment.

Translated from the French text, this volume provides case studies and examples from the author's art psychotherapy practice of 40 years, including the 'four-quadrants method'. Chapters review the current treatments for chronic pain and post-traumatic stress disorder (PTSD) and focus on art therapeutic methods to treat those conditions, such as art therapy protocols for PTSD. The book exposes the underlying rational of somatic art therapy, covering art therapy effectiveness, Levine's somatic dissociation, van der Kolk's somatic memory, and Scaer's procedural memory concepts. Also featured are chapter contributions from art therapists Sophie Boudrias, Mylène Piché, and Dr. Patcharin Sughondhabirom.

By providing a unique, clear, and concise synthesis of available art therapy methods, this text will appeal both to the general and professional public, including professional art therapists, psychotherapists, helping relation professionals, and medical practitioners.

**Johanne Hamel**, Doctor in Psychology, psychologist, and art psychotherapist, specializes in Somatic art therapy as well as in dreamwork and art therapy. She is an international lecturer in Canada, Europe, the USA, and Thailand.

**Hélène Hamel** is a self-employed translator who holds an Honors degree in translation and has worked mainly on translation from English to French for more than 30 years.

'3 words for Johanne Hamel "**Sweet**", "**Deep**" and "**Original**".

3 words for this book of hers "A MUST", "A MUST" and "A MUST" as well as "**Fulfilling**".

It's like reading a love story in which there are multiple encounters between "Theory" and "Practice". Johanne Hamel is extremely successful in creating a connection between "Theory" and "Practice", using her own examples from her art psychotherapy practice of many years.'

Jo Sughondhabirom, MD, RCAT, International
Program of Art Therapy in Thailand

'Johanne Hamel has expanded the healing potential of Art Therapy by incorporating somatic processing, providing her students and clients with the opportunity to gain a deeper awareness about the mind-body connection in emotional healing and wellbeing. As a somatic art therapist, Johanne Hamel developed a 6-days intensive workshop in *Somatic Art Therapy* and now she has provided us with this valuable text on Somatic art therapy, first published in French and now in English. Although, releasing trauma from the body may not be a new concept in the field of mental health, blending art therapy interventions with somatic processing in trauma treatment is a promising new concept in the field of Art Therapy.'

From the Foreword, Lucille Proulx, MA, ATR, RCAT,
executive director, CiiAT- The Canadian International
Institute of Art Therapy.

# Somatic Art Therapy

Alleviating Pain and Trauma through Art

Johanne Hamel

**Translated by**
**Hélène Hamel**

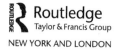
Routledge
Taylor & Francis Group

NEW YORK AND LONDON

First published 2021
by Routledge
52 Vanderbilt Avenue, New York, NY 10017

and by Routledge
2 Park Square, Milton Park, Abingdon, Oxon OX14 4RN

*Routledge is an imprint of the Taylor & Francis Group, an informa business*

Originally published in French as:

L'art-thérapie somatique. Pour aider à guérir la douleur chronique.

*Library of Congress Cataloging-in-Publication Data*
Names: Hamel, Johanne, 1952- author.
Title: Somatic art therapy : alleviating pain and trauma
through art / Johanne Hamel.
Description: New York : Routledge, 2021. |
Includes bibliographical references and index. |
Identifiers: LCCN 2020048600 (print) | LCCN 2020048601 (ebook) |
ISBN 9780367903244 (hardback) | ISBN 9780367903244 (paperback) |
ISBN 9781003023746 (ebook)
Subjects: LCSH: Pain--Treatment. | Art therapy.
Classification: LCC RB127 .H328 2021 (print) | LCC RB127 (ebook) |
DDC 615.8/5156--dc23
LC record available at https://lccn.loc.gov/2020048600
LC ebook record available at https://lccn.loc.gov/2020048601

ISBN: 978-0-367-90324-4 (hbk)
ISBN: 978-0-367-90323-7 (pbk)
ISBN: 978-1-003-02374-6 (ebk)

Typeset in Times New Roman
by Taylor & Francis Books

This book is dedicated to all traumatized children, women and men, especially from sexual abuse of any kind

# Contents

*List of figures*     xi
*Foreword*     xiv
*Acknowledgements*     xv
*List of abbreviations*     xvi
*List of contributors*     xvii

Introduction     1

**PART I**
**Definitions**     5

1   Somatic Art Therapy     7

*A brief history of humanist art therapy 7*
*Definition of somatic art therapy 8*
*The limits of somatic art therapy 9*

2   Chronic Pain     10

*Acute pain, chronic pain and suffering, a distinction 10*
*Currently known treatments for chronic pain 11*

3   Post-Traumatic Stress Disorder (PTSD)     14

*Definition of post-traumatic stress disorder (PTSD) 14*

**PART II**
**An Overview of Art Therapy Treatments: An Overview**     23

4   Art Therapy for PTSD and Chronic Pain: An Overview     25

*Art therapy treatments for chronic pain: Examples 25*
*Art therapy and PTSD 27*
*Art therapy protocols for PTSD treatments 29*

5  Trauma Treatment: Eight Techniques for Art Therapists          32

*Abreaction techniques 32*
*Motor reaction de-freezing techniques 33*
*Intense emotional expression techniques 33*
*Affect restoration techniques 35*
*Stress reduction and relaxation techniques 36*
*Safe haven techniques 36*
*Identity reconstruction techniques 36*
*Personal integrity restoration techniques 37*

**PART III**
**Theoretical Concepts**                                          39

6  Hypotheses About Art Therapy Effectiveness                     41

*The power of images to facilitate abreaction 41*
*Right brain stimulation 42*
*Isomorphism 42*
*Objectification 43*
*Containment 44*
*Security 44*

7  Dissociative Processes in Post-Traumatic Stress Disorders      46

*Levine's somatic dissociation: The SIBAM model 46*
*Van der Kolk's somatic memory 47*
*Scaer's procedural memory 49*

8  Neuroscience and Somatic Art Therapy: Emotional Memory
   Reconsolidation                                                51

*Emotional memory 51*
*Memory consolidation and reconsolidation 52*
*Emotional avoidance 52*
*The prerequisites in psychotherapy 53*
*Identifying the symptom 53*
*Identifying a symptom: case example 54*
*Identifying the schema 55*

*Symptom amplification: case example 56*
*Symptom deprivation: case example 58*
*Identifying or creating a counter-experience 60*
*Counter-experience: case example 60*
*Facilitating the emotional memory reconsolidation process 62*

9  Somatic Heart Coherence and the Quantum Model            63

*Connection with our source design 64*
*The heart as an intuitive brain 65*
*Experiential method: somatic heart coherence. Restoring the*
*    connection with the overlooked brain 67*
*Case study: The reunification 67*
*The quantum power of self-love 73*
*Understanding intuitive intelligence 74*
*Conclusion 77*

**PART IV**
**Somatic Art Therapy Applications**                        81

10  Somatic Art Therapy Intervention Methods for Chronic Pain   83

*The four-quadrants method 83*
*Hands-on healing 84*
*Small silhouette drawing 85*
*Life-size silhouette 86*
*Art process therapy 86*

11  'Four-quadrants' Method Case Studies                     88

*Case study A 89*
*Case study B 93*
*Case study C 97*
*Case study D 101*
*Case study E 107*

12  Somatic Art Therapy and Chronic Pain: Case Studies       114

*Case study A: Back pain following a motor vehicle accident –*
*    access to procedural memory 114*
*Case study B: A brief example of whiplash symptoms 118*
*Case story C: Acquired dyspareunia, a process art*
*    psychotherapy treatment 120*

## 13   A Healing Metaphor                                             123

*First day of the workshop: The life-size silhouette 123*
*Second day of the workshop: The 'four-quadrants' method 126*
*Third day of the workshop: A giant scribble 130*
*Fourth day of the workshop: Exploring a burning sensation 131*
*Fifth day of the workshop: A healing metaphor 133*

Conclusion: The Importance of Developing Somatic Art Therapy
Research                                                              142

*Appendices*                                                          144
*Appendix A*                                                          145
*Appendix B*                                                          153
*Appendix C*                                                          155
*Bibliography*                                                        159
*Author's index*                                                      170
*Subject index*                                                       171

# Figures

8.1    The symptom, 12 inches x 18 inches (30.5 cm x 45 cm). Oil pastels, soft pastel, and coloured pencils. Pressure and vibration at the contact boundary. The arrow and the heart shape were added during the process    55

8.2    Amplification of the symptom, 8½ inches x 11 inches (21.6 cm x 28 cm). Oil pastels, coloured pencils, and gouache. The arrow that is cutting through and the void within the black line were added during the process    57

8.3    The symptom: the tags, 18 inches x 24 inches (45 cm x 60 cm). Coloured pencils and oil pastels. The cutting out, the purple circle around the character, and the blue circle inside were added during the process    58

8.4    Symptom deprivation: Letting go of the tags. 18 inches x 24 inches (45 cm x 60 cm). Colored pencils and oil pastels    59

8.5    Counter-experience: the snail recharging in nature (cross-sectional view), about 6 inches x 8 inches (15 cm x 20 cm). Clay    61

9.1    Emily's silhouette, before the introduction of *somatic heart coherence*, 5 feet x 7 feet (152 cm x 215 cm), chalk pastels and gouache    68

9.2    Emily's representation of the heart soma (part one), 5 feet x 5 feet, 152 cm x 152 cm, color pencils    69

9.3    Emily's representation of her heart soma, with the *hands-on healing* method (part two), 5 feet x 5 feet (152 cm x 152 cm), color pencils and gouache. On the bottom: the completed image, 5 feet x 5 feet (152 cm x 152 cm), colour pencils and gouache    71

11.1    (First drawing, quadrant #1) *The pain.* 18 inches x 24 inches (45 cm x 60 cm). Oil pastels    89

11.2    (Second drawing, quadrant #2) *The past origin of the pain.* 18 inches x 24 inches (45 cm x 60 cm). Felt tips    90

11.3    (Third drawing, quadrant #4) *Healing.* 18 inches x 24 inches (45 cm x 60 cm). Oil pastels    91

11.4    (Fourth drawing, quadrant #3) *Transition to healing.* 18 inches x 24 inches (45 cm x 60 cm). Oil pastels and watercolours                                                                92

11.5    (First drawing, quadrant #1) *The sensation.* 18 inches x 24 inches (45 cm x 60 cm). Tempera. (Reproduction)                       93

11.6    (Second drawing, quadrant #2) *The past experience.* 18 inches x 24 inches (45 cm x 60 cm). Tempera. (Reproduction)                                                                94

11.7    (Third drawing, quadrant #4) *Healing of shoulder blades.* 18 inches x 24 inches (45 x 60 cm). Tempera. (Reproduction)                                                                95

11.8    (Fourth drawing, quadrant #3) *The transition.* 18 inches x 24 inches (45 cm x 60 cm). Tempera. (Reproduction)                   96

11.9    (First drawing, quadrant #1) *Drawing the discomfort.* 18 inches x 24 inches (45 cm x 60 cm). Tempera                       97

11.10   (Second drawing, quadrant #2) *The imprisoned anger.* About 15 inches x 15 inches (about 38 cm x 38 cm). Tempera                                                                        98

11.11   (Third drawing, quadrant #4) *Healing.* About 15 inches x 15 inches (about 38 cm x 38 cm). Tempera                       99

11.12   (Fourth drawing, quadrant #3) *The transition.* About 15 inches x 15 inches (about 38 cm x 38 cm). Tempera           100

11.13   (First drawing, quadrant #1) *The painful sensation.* About 15 inches x 15 inches (about 38 cm x 38 cm). Tempera      102

11.14   (Second drawing, quadrant #2) *The past.* About 15 inches x 15 inches (about 38 cm x 38 cm). Tempera              103

11.15   (Third drawing, quadrant #4) *The healing.* About 15 inches x 15 inches (about 38 cm x 38 cm). Tempera              104

11.16   (Fourth drawing, quadrant #3) *The transition.* About 15 inches x 15 inches (about 38 cm x 38 cm). Tempera           106

11.17   The four-quadrants mandala. 5 feet x 5 feet (1.52 m x 1.52 m). Tempera                                                           107

11.18   The fragmented body. 5 feet x 8 feet (1.52 m x 2.44 m). Mix media                                                                 108

11.19   The four-quadrants mandala. 5 feet x 5 feet (1.52 m x 1.52 m). Mix media                                                         110

11.20   Pippa Longstocking, the Bad Girl on the block or Little Pest. 5 feet x 5 feet (1.52 m x 1.52 m). Drawing pencils and oil pastels                                                           111

11.21   The left side pain. 5 feet x 5 feet (1.52 m x 1.52 m). Oil pastels                                                                 112

12.1    (First drawing, first session) *The pain.* 18 inches x 24 inches (45 cm x 60 cm). Dry pastels                               115

12.2    (Second drawing, first session) *The pain amplified.* 18 inches x 24 inches (45 cm x 60 cm). Dry pastels                 116

| | | |
|---|---|---|
| 12.3 | (First drawing, second session) *The location of pain.* 18 inches x 24 inches (45 cm x 60 cm). Dry pastels | 117 |
| 12.4 | (Second drawing, second session) *The pain amplified and pressure exerted.* 18 inches x 24 inches (45 cm x 60 cm). Dry pastels | 117 |
| 12.5 | *The shoulder pain.* 18 inches x 24 inches (45 cm x 60 cm). Oil pastels | 119 |
| 12.6 | *The knot at the core of the pain.* 18 inches x 24 inches (45 cm x 60 cm). Oil pastels | 119 |
| 12.7 | *Lines within the pain knot.* 18 inches x 24 inches (45 cm x 60 cm). Oil pastels | 120 |
| 13.1 | *The silhouette.* 34 inches x 80 inches (85 cm x 195 cm). Mixed media, tempera on 50 pounds (80 g/m) paper, cotton pads and, sewing threads | 124 |
| 13.2 | Details of the right foot | 125 |
| 13.3 | Details of the calf | 126 |
| 13.4 | The four quadrants, 44 inches x 58 inches (110 cm x 145 cm). Oil pastels on 100 pounds (160 g/m) drawing paper | 128 |
| 13.5A | *The hourglass shape.* 34 inches x 34 inches (75 cm x 75 cm). Pencil on 50 pounds (80 g/m) paper | 130 |
| 13.5B | *The stable hourglass shape.* 34 inches x 34 inches (75 cm x 75 cm). Mixed media including acrylic paints and oil pastels | 130 |
| 13.6 | *The burning sensation.* 24 inches x 29 inches (60 cm x 82½ cm). Oil pastels on 100 pounds (160 g/m) drawing paper | 131 |
| 13.7 | The three layers of the body on the floor | 134 |
| 13.8 | The 'operating table' | 135 |
| 13.9 | The body on the 'operating table' | 136 |
| 13.10 | Repositioning of the arms and reconstruction of the shoulders | 138 |
| 13.11 | Application of the new born skin colour and environment colours. 34 inches x 80 inches (85 cm x 195 cm). Mixed media including 50 pounds (80 g/m) white paper, 112 pounds (180 g/m) brown paper, acrylic paints, TOA Latex glue | 139 |

# Foreword

The magic of imagery and the understanding of the transformative potential of the art-making process is the profession of art therapists. This transformative process occurs in the context of the relationship between the client, the image, and the therapist. Johanne Hamel has expanded the healing potential of art therapy by incorporating somatic processing, providing her students and clients with the opportunity to gain a deeper awareness about the mind-body connection in emotional healing and wellbeing.

As a somatic art therapist, Johanne Hamel has dedicated her career to promoting and growing the profession of art therapy, first in Québec, in 1995, as founder of the Institut de formation professionnelle en psychothérapie par l'art, in Sherbrooke, Québec, Canada, creating the first French art therapy training program. She also developed her six-day intensive workshop 'Art as Medicine', and now Johanne has provided us with this valuable text on somatic art therapy, first published in French and now in English. Although releasing trauma from the body might not be a new concept in the field of mental health, blending art therapy interventions with somatic processing in trauma treatment is a promising new concept in the field of art therapy.

As an established art therapist, attachment specialist in the field for over 35 years, the director of an International Art Therapy Institute, and a colleague of Johanne Hamel for over 20 years, I have witnessed the profession go through many transformations, but this "psychosomatic" work is crucial to the continuous enhancement and development in the field of art therapy. I am grateful to Johanne for sharing her wisdom and ongoing enthusiasm for somatic art therapy as she trains art therapists and mental health professionals in Canada, Central America, Europe, and Asia.

Lucille Proulx, MA, ATR, RCAT, Executive Director, The Canadian International Institute of Art Therapy

# Acknowledgements

I would especially like to acknowledge three special contributors to this edition, who are all esteemed colleagues of mine: Dr. Sophie Boudrias, PsyD, ATPQ, art psychotherapist; Mylène Piché, MA, ATPQ, art therapist; and Dr. Patcharin Sughondhabirom, MD, RCAT, and art therapist. It is a pleasure to work with you all, and I am very grateful for your very knowledgeable contributions. You are helping readers to understand even more deeply the wisdom of somatic art therapy.

My deepest and heartfelt gratefulness to Lucille Proulx, MA, ATR, RCAT, art therapist, attachment specialist in the field of art therapy for over 35 years, and director of the Canadian International Institute of Art Therapy and my personal mentor, for your unwavering support all those years since we have known each other.

Also, many thanks to my sister, Hélène Hamel. You relentlessly searched for the most meaningful ways to express our thoughts in all their nuances, and I appreciate that very much.

Johanne Hamel, D. Ps., RCAT

# List of abbreviations

ATPQ: Professional member of the Québec Art Therapy Association
ATR: Professional member of the American Art Therapy Association
CATA: Canadian Art Therapy Association
CIIAT: Canadian International Institute of Art Therapy
D. Ps.: Doctoral degree in psychology
DSM-V: Diagnostic and statistical manual of mental disorders, no. 5
EMDR: Eye movement desensitization and reprocessing
IPATT: International Program of Art Therapy in Thailand
MA: Master's degree
MD: Doctor in medicine
MR: Memory reconsolidation
MVA: Motor vehicle accident
PsyD: Doctoral degree in Psychology
PTSD: Post-traumatic stress disorder
RCAT: Registered Professional member of the canadian Art therapy Association

# Contributors

**Johanne Hamel, D. Ps., ATPQ, RCAT, psychologist, and art psychotherapist**

**Author of all chapters except chapters 8, 9, and 13 and editor of contributed chapters.**

**Johanne Hamel**, psychologist and art psychotherapist, specializes in Somatic art therapy as well as in Dreamwork and art therapy. She has been teaching art therapy for twenty years at Université du Québec en Abitibi-Témiscamingue, Québec, Canada. She has published three books in art therapy in French, including a co-authored book on art therapy with Larousse, Paris, and has published *Art therapy, Dreams and Healing. Beyond the looking Glass,* with Routledge in 2021. She is currently an international lecturer in Thailand, in the USA at the International Association for the Study of Dreams and in Europe, for the European Consortium for Art Therapies Education. She maintains a private practice in Sherbrooke, Québec, Canada.

**Dr. Sophie Boudrias, PsyD, ATPQ, art psychotherapist**

**Chapter 8: Neuroscience and Somatic Art Therapy: Emotional Memory Reconsolidation**

**Sophie Boudrias** is a psychologist and art psychotherapist. She specializes in humanistic and emotion-centered approaches, as well as in emotional memory reconsolidation, dream work, and process work. As a member of a crisis unit, she conducted several individual and group post-traumatic interventions. She also leads conferences on various topics related to her profession, such as self-awareness and art therapy. She is the author of the French book "Create your own legend" (Créez votre légende personnelle) and the creator of a projective art therapy assessment tool, called Draw-a-Wild-Animal-and-a-Person. She currently teaches art therapy at Université du Québec en Abitibi-Témiscamingue, Québec, Canada.

**Mylène Piché, MA, ATPQ, artist and art therapist**

**Chapter 9: Somatic Heart Coherence and the Quantum Model**

**Mylène Piché, M.A. ATPQ**, artist and art therapist, currently teaches art therapy in the Master's degree program at Université du Québec en Abitibi-Témiscamingue. Her focus of expertise, is at the crossroads of quantum healing, body awareness, and artistic expression as a therapeutic modality. She specializes in the field of somatic coherence as she applies quantum principles to the creative process.

**Dr. Patcharin Sughondhabirom, MD, RCAT, art therapist**

**Chapter 13: A Healing Metaphor**

**Dr. Patcharin Sughondhabirom** (also known as Dr. Jo) is a medical doctor and registered art therapist who lives in Bangkok, Thailand. In 2005 she started an open art studio project for children with cancer at the King Chulalongkorn Memorial Hospital and the Queen Sirikit Institute of Children's Health in Bangkok. In 2011 she started a collaboration with the Canadian International Institute of Art Therapy and developed The International Program of Art Therapy in Thailand. She is regularly invited to speak and give lectures at academic institutions and universities around the country and has written a number of books and contributed chapters on the subject of art therapy with children in palliative care.

Note on the translator:

**Hélène Hamel** is a self-employed translator who holds an Honor degree in translation and has been working mainly on translations from English to French for more than 30 years. She occasionally accepts translation work from French to English. Over the years, she has developed a great interest in therapy practices and alternative medicine, and she is now focussing on the publishing world.

# Introduction

*Johanne Hamel*

I have been working on chronic and acute pain for the last 35 years, since the day when I designed a six-day intensive workshop in Somatic art therapy, which I taught at least 20 times at Université du Québec en Abitibi-Témiscamingue, in Québec, Canada. Through my work, I was able to discover and confirm the value of somatic art therapy as a means to get a clear understanding of the psychological meaning of a physical pain and to achieve pain relief and sometimes even to completely eliminate a specific pain. So I am extremely pleased to present the findings of this empirical research.

Let me introduce three very special contributors who have accepted to write a new chapter for this English version of the book *L'art-thérapie somatique*, which was first published in French. Their contributions add very meaningful concepts and case stories, and the book benefits wonderfully from their knowledge and wisdom. These contributors are Dr. Sophie Boudrias, PsyD, ATPQ, art psychotherapist; Mylène Piché, MA, ATPQ, art therapist; and Dr. Patcharin Sughondhabirom, MD, RCAT, medical doctor and art therapist, all estimated colleagues of mine.

This practical guide is intended firstly for professional art therapists, as they are knowledgeable about the art therapy tools presented here, especially if they are trained in art process therapy.[1]

However, this guide is also designed to appeal both to the general and professional public, including psychotherapists, help relationship professionals and medical practitioners, and we hope to bring a sense of how psyche and states of consciousness influence disease and healing. As Dr. Andrew Weil[2] states, while Asclepius, the God of medicine in ancient Greece, used medicinal procedures like surgery and drugs, his daughter, Hygieia, Goddess of health, prevention and healing, achieved healing from within by drawing on the human body's inherent healing physical and psychological capacities, which are always available. Dr. Weil envisions the future development of Western medicine as increasingly integrating these two forces.

Western medicine would also benefit from understanding the heart–brain mechanisms and influence on the body. Art therapist Mylène Piché, MA,

ATPQ, provides insights in Chapter 9 about how the heart's somatic coherence is an essential component of our overall balance and helps the reader to understand the role that it plays in the attainment of healing states of consciousness. The author also discusses the contribution of quantum physics to our current medical model and looks at how it is possible to use somatic art therapy to improve access to our own quantum healing potentials. As various states of consciousness are revealed to have a crucial influence in the manifestation of disease and health, she invites us to look at healing processes beyond physical matter, into the quantum field and the energetic design that is created by our emotions and our thought patterns. Which is exactly what we do in somatic art therapy.

My hope is also to promote recognition of the specific contribution of art therapists, who deserve to find their place in the healthcare system and to be increasingly recognized for the unique services that they can offer. This book will hopefully provide you with valuable insight in this area.

The approaches presented in this book might be self-facilitated. However, applying the art therapy methods presented in chapter 10 is only recommended if you are accustomed to working on yourself. The reasons behind this word of caution will be specified in chapter 10. Nonetheless, my recommendation is to use these approaches in the safe context of a structured relationship with a professional art therapist or art psychotherapist.

This book has four different parts and focuses on somatic art therapy for treating chronic pain, especially resulting from physical and/or psychological trauma.

In **Part 1: Definitions,** after introducing art therapy, somatic art therapy, and the current knowledge about chronic pain in chapters 1 and 2, a definition of post-traumatic stress disorders (PTSD) will be provided based on the DSM V[3], followed by explanations about the typical treatments for these disorders, as well as the relationship between PTSD and chronic pain, which feature in chapter 3.

**Part 2: An overview of art therapy treatments** expands on known art therapy treatments. Art therapists have developed a fairly substantive body of knowledge and a great deal of expertise about treatments for PTSD and dissociative states (which are central in PTSD) and about chronic pain, to a lesser degree. So in Chapter 4 I made sure to provide an overview of the literature on art therapy and to summarize the various intervention procedures applied to all kinds of traumatic situations. Chapter 5 presents eight types of techniques used in art therapeutic intervention procedures that are relevant to trauma treatment. Therefore, this book can also appeal to those interested in the treatment of trauma and PTSD through art therapy, whether there is pain or not.

**Part 3: Theoretical concepts** looks at the theoretical foundations likely to explain how effective art therapy is for treating trauma treatment and chronic pain. Chapter 6 summarizes six hypotheses about art therapy effectiveness. Chapter 7 focuses on three authors on the subject of dissociative processes, which are very important in PTSD: Levine (2005, 2009, 2015), van der Kolk (1987, 1994, 1996, 1998), and Scaer (2001). Knowledge about those processes allows for effective somatic art therapy interventions. Sophie Boudrias, PSYD, ATPQ, art psychotherapist and author of chapter 8 *Neuroscience and somatic art therapy*, focuses on emotional memory reconsolidation, which is a basic concept in neuroscience that will help the reader to understand the effectiveness of art therapy methods and techniques in activating emotional memories, so that they can be transformed. This chapter aims to illustrate and provide insights into the specific contribution of art therapy, especially of somatic art therapy, in order to facilitate the emotional memory reconsolidation process. The mobilization of the body in the act of creating, as well as the properties of the image, the metaphor, and the creative process constitute powerful therapeutic levers, both to reveal emotional memories and to transform them. Chapter 9 covers the somatic heart coherence and quantum model that I mentioned above.

Finally, **Part 4: Somatic art therapy applications** covers many examples of somatic art therapy interventions, with clients suffering from a variety of different physical afflictions. Chapter 10 describes four specific somatic art therapy methods for chronic pain, including the 'four-quadrants method', and chapters 11 to 13 include examples and case studies demonstrating how valuable, relevant, and efficient these methods can be.

Let me especially introduce chapter 13 written by Dr. Patcharin Sughondhabirom, MD, RCAT, art therapist from Thailand, or Dr. Jo, as we affectionately call her! Dr. Jo, while assisting me in a somatic art therapy workshop in Thailand, offered to apply her medical knowledge to a somatic art therapy intervention in helping a student suffering from severe chronic pains. Although I was not sure at first that it could be done, I suddenly understood the brilliant metaphor that she was thinking about and agreed for her to conduct this special intervention. It took about three hours. The results were unbelievable: it became one of the most powerful moments of healing that I witnessed in my whole career – a really sacred moment. As you will see in the pictures, the room that she was working in felt like a real operating room. The other students and I were in awe and kept silent at times during our own work, as we felt that we were witnessing something very special happening before our very eyes. Afterwards, Dr. Jo said that she had never felt prouder of being a medical doctor while doing this somatic art therapy intervention. So, I insisted that Dr. Jo write about her very special intervention, and that is what you will find in chapter 13. It is very endearing that through her English words, we can see her Thai culture coming through.

We hope at the end of these presentations that you will emerge with a strong sense of the importance of psyche and of the heart–brain connection in healing, and, just as importantly, that you will be able to envision the possible contribution of art therapists in a modern healthcare system, which would capture their specificity, their relevance, and their importance.

## Notes

1 See Chapter 1 for a brief explanation of this approach and also Rhinehart, L. & Engelhorn, P. (1982), 'Pre-image considerations as a therapeutic process'. *The Arts in Psychotherapy*, 9, pp. 55–63.
2 Weil, Andrew. Doctor and author of *Spontaneous Healing: How to discover and enhance your body's natural ability to maintain and heal itself.* Kindle Edition, 2014.
3 See Appendix 1 for an excerpt from the American Psychiatric Association (2013). Mini-Desk Reference to the Diagnostic Criteria from the DSM-V. Washington, DC: APA.

# Part I
# Definitions

# 1 Somatic Art Therapy

*Johanne Hamel*

Art therapy is a form of psychotherapeutic intervention that uses the visual arts as a medium of expression. Far from being offered solely to artists, art therapy uses intervention tools such as lines, forms, colors in drawings, paintings, assemblage, or collage, which make it a practice accessible to all types of clientele. Art therapists are trained in both psychology and art before they are trained in art therapy.

## A brief history of humanist art therapy

Art therapy is very recent in historical terms. In Europe first and then in the USA, the artists hired to provide activities for psychiatric patients soon realized how their action had psychotherapeutic effects, and they began to observe and scientifically document their interventions. Several professional journals were launched, and there is now a growing wealth of specialized literature on the subject. As artists had to turn to psychoanalytically oriented psychiatrists for the most part, nearly all of the art therapists trained in psychoanalysis, and most of them are currently using the psychoanalytic intervention rationale to explain their action. Some, however, use the Jungian approach, the object relations approach, the Adlerian or Kleinian approach, while others use a humanistic approach.

It was not until the 1970s[1] that Janie Rhyne (1973) introduced the Gestalt approach to art therapy based on the humanist perspective. Even more innovative, in the 1980s Rhinehart and Engelhorn[2] (1982) developed the *Art process therapy*, using a combination of the Gestalt and Jungian approaches in their intervention rationale. Instead of limiting themselves to considering only the finished artwork, Rhinehart and Engelhorn also use amplification of lines, shapes, colors, and movements as they emerge on paper to explore them thoroughly in order to bring out the inherent and unexpected psychological meaning. Art therapists specializing in the *Art process therapy* approach consider observation of the process as the main source of their intervention, while leaving it to the client to figure out the meaning, given that she/he is the expert on her/his own experience. This is a typically humanist perspective.

In Québec, Canada, many French-speaking art therapists were trained in this approach, first at the Institut de formation professionnelle en psychothérapie par l'art between 1995 and 2005, where the two main professors had been taught by Rhinehart and Engelhorn[3], then at the Université du Québec en Abitibi-Témiscamingue, where the *Art therapy process* approach is taught and where programs have been developed since 1997. Concordia University was the first to offer an art therapy Master's degree in Québec, Canada, in 1980, and its approach is mainly psychoanalytical.

Art therapists offer a unique and indispensable contribution to all clients who cannot express themselves through verbal language or whose privileged mode of expression is not language, such as children or First Nations people. However, they also deal with all the clients that psychologists, psychotherapists, and counselors are likely to encounter: psychiatric patients; teens with behavior problems; elderly people with cognitive losses; women experiencing violence or sexual abuse; community settings offering a wide range of services to all kinds of clienteles; persons with cancer and their families; persons undergoing bereavement, burnout, divorce or separation; and hospitalized children, as well as many others.

## Definition of somatic art therapy

The somatic art therapy approach outlined here stems from my knowledge and my experience in art therapy, and mainly from Levine, van der Kolk, and Scaer's theories, three authors who wrote on post-traumatic stress disorders and their dissociative states (See chapter 7). Somatic art therapy refers to the interventions and therapeutic tools that I have intuitively developed over the past 30 years.

Rinfret (2000) defines the term *soma* as follows, distinguishing it from the body:

"The term *body* refers to the physical reality of human beings as perceived by an outsider, whereas the word *soma* represents that same physical reality as it is experienced from within the person" (p. 44) (Free translation).

So it is a matter of subjectively feeling the inner reality and apprehending it phenomenologically. My own definition of somatic art therapy therefore is the following: somatic art therapy provides access to soma through two-dimensional or three-dimensional representations (drawing, painting, clay, etc.) of the physical sensation felt subjectively. This access makes one aware of intense emotional states embedded in one's sensations, allows catharsis and facilitates communication of these experiences.

My methods have many affinities with Levine's somatic experiencing (SE)[4]. SE uses the felt sense to access the traumatic response, concentrating deliberately on the intricacies of the somatic sensation. This is exactly what we do in somatic art therapy, because drawing the physical sensation requires paying attention to all its proprioceptive manifestations. Through drawing or painting, the patient gains access to the *somatic procedural memory*, an expression proposed by Scaer[5] for traumatic memories stored in the right brain, implicated in the perpetuation of some traumatic reactions.[6] Finally, somatic art therapy relies on Rhinehart and Engelhorn's art process therapy approach[7], which in turn rests on Gestalt and Jungian theoretical rationales and on Humanist psychology. To develop this approach, I applied art process therapy to soma work. In Part 3 of this book, the theoretical bases of art therapy and of somatic art therapy will be explained further.

## The limits of somatic art therapy

I typically use somatic art therapy to work on distressing pain or physical sensations, in individual encounters which are part of a broader psychotherapeutic process or in intensive six-day workshop context conducive to deep inner work. The *temenos* [8] is obviously crucial for a successful intervention, as for any psychotherapeutic process.

Furthermore, I learned from experience that somatic art therapy works better on specific pains located in definite body areas. With respect to dull pain, such as in fibromyalgia or chronic fatigue, a long-term art psychotherapeutic journey might be appropriate, in addition to other types of interventions such as dietary changes, regular physical exercise, etc.

In some cases of chronic pain, the intervention must be long-term, as in the example of acquired dyspareunia presented in chapter 12 (C). In terms of diseases, more extensive research will be required to better apprehend how somatic art therapy could support treatment, besides interventions on the painful sensations as such.

## Notes

1 Rhyne, J. (1973). *The Gestalt Art Experience*. Pacific Grove, CA: Brooks/Cole Publishing Co.
2 Rhinehart, L. & Engelhorn, P. (1982), 'Pre-image considerations as a therapeutic process'. *The Arts in Psychotherapy*, 9, 55–63.
3 At the Eagle Rock Trail Art Therapy Institute in Santa Rosa, California, initially affiliated with Sonoma State University, then separated from it.
4 Levine, P. (1997). *Waking the Tiger*. Berkeley, CA: North Atlantic Press.
5 Scaer, P. (2001). *The Body Bears the Burden, Trauma, Dissociation, and Disease*. Binghamton, NY: The Haworth Medical Press.
6 For an example of this phenomenon, see the case study included in Chapter 11 (A).
7 Rhinehart, L. and Engelhorn, P. (1982): *Op. Cit.*
8 Duchastel, A. (2005). *La voie de l'imaginaire. Le processus en art-thérapie*. Montréal, Qc.: Quebecor.

# 2   Chronic Pain

*Johanne Hamel*

## Acute pain, chronic pain and suffering, a distinction

There are many different types of pains. Very important distinctions need to be made for understanding the subject. The International Association for the Study of Pain[1] defines pain as 'an unpleasant sensory and emotional experience associated with, or resembling that associated with, actual or potential tissue damage', chronic pain exceeding a criterion of six months. Acute pain is defined as short-term pain that lasts less than six months and is a predictable response to an injury or illness. Its intensity is also predictable. Chronic pain can also be a pain that has been going on for a short while, but is more intense than what is usually expected for a particular injury or illness. Chronic pain can be continuous or intermittent. The Association believes that pain is always a very personal experience and when reported by an individual, it should always be respected.

Researchers have found that there is no adequate medical explanation in most cases of chronic pain; the percentages reported vary greatly in studies and can go up to 85% of cases where the pain cannot be explained from a medical point of view.[2]

Chronic pain brings a whole range of psychological and psychosocial problems, including anxiety, depression, unemployment, marital tensions, suicide, disability, and psychological distress.[3]

It seems more and more accepted that a bio-psycho-social model gives a better understanding of chronic pain than a bio-medical model: it is now clear that the cause of pain is not exclusively biological (resulting from physical impairment) or exclusively psychological, as previously thought.[4] Chronic pain rather involves complex and interrelated mechanisms at all levels in a person's life.

The distinction between pain and suffering allows us to better understand that point. Suffering is a much more global process, involving the whole person in her psychological, moral, and even spiritual aspects. Dr. Beauchamp considers that:

'Physical pain in chronic diseases is always the starting point of a suffering process which is a mingling of the tangible body and the intangible soul, of the experience of the patient, the family teachings, the spiritual ideas he adhered to, his friends, his occupation, the grudges he is bearing, the regrets about what could have been or remorse for having committed the wrong. The patient going through physical and moral pain is suffering a lot. His pain must be eased and relief is needed for why it hurts so much'.[5]

### *Chronic pain prevalence*

Chronic pain is extremely widespread. In Canada, three out of ten people are suffering from it, and there are more women and people aged 50 or older who live with it.[6] People suffer from back pain (35%), leg pain (21%), headaches (15%), neck pain (14%), etc.; pain can actually affect any part of the body or joints in general.[7] In addition, about 70% to 80% of adults will suffer from chronic pain at some point in their lives.[8] Chronic pain is actually the most common complaint of patients to their health professionals. In the USA, it is estimated to account for trillion of dollars a year in productivity losses and healthcare costs.[9]

Countless studies[10] indicate a co-occurrence of chronic pain and post-traumatic stress disorder (PTSD), both in patients consulting for chronic pain and those consulting for PTSD. In fact, those consulting for PSTD even have the highest co-prevalence rates. These results are consistent for both veterans and those consulting for work-related injuries as well as for motor vehicle accident victims, patients with fibromyalgia, and burn vic-tims. For example, a large majority of 129 Vietnam War veterans (80%) reported having chronic pain, in a self-administered questionnaire to assess symptoms of PTSD and pain.[11]

In a literature review, it was found that more than 25% of patients seeking treatment for chronic pain and substance abuse suffer from PTSD[12] and vice versa; another study found a prevalence of about 10% to 35% of PTSD in cases of chronic pain.[13]

To give a better idea of the very high prevalence of chronic pain, a good example might be the whiplash effect. The whiplash syndrome usually develops as a result of a rear-end car collision or a sudden change in speed in an accident involving some other means of transportation.[14] The whiplash symptoms are neck pain, rigidity, and sensitivity; in addition, possible mus-culoskeletal signs of decreased range of motion and sensitivity at specific points can occur in more severe cases. There are more than one million acute whiplash injuries a year in the USA and one-third of injured Americans still experience chronic whiplash symptoms 33 months after the accident.[15]

## Currently known treatments for chronic pain

As it is currently recognized that chronic pain is a psycho-bio-social phenomenon, it is considered that the best treatment approach is multi-disciplinary and includes psychological treatment.[16] This means that treatment will include drugs to manage pain as much as possible, that psychotherapy will also be recommended and that the quality and extent of the supportive social network will also be taken into account. It seems an adequate social support system will decrease the perception of pain.

Camic uses Melzack and Wall's[17] gate control theory to explain chronic pain:

The gate is controlled by both transmission from the site of injury and from transmissions from the brain. The messages from the brain (which are referred to as afferent and descending tract messages) are presumed to be influenced by emotional and cognitive factors. If these factors cause the gate to open, there will be a perception of increased pain. If, on the other hand, the messages allow the gate to close, there will be a decrease in pain perception.[18] For Camic, this theory points to the need to use a large range of interventions, in particular the cognitive-behavioral approach:

In the biopsychosocial treatment of pain, cognitive behavioral approaches to pain management have been widely accepted as preferred methods of treatment when emotional, behavioral, cognitive, and/or social factors exacerbate pain.[19]

Specialized literature is in general agreement with him: indeed, most of the treatments used for chronic pain currently derive from cognitive behavioral approaches, so far.[20]

## Notes

1   International Association for the Study of Pain. www.iasp-pain.org, accessed September 7, 2020.
2   Seyo *et al.*, 1991, cited in Grant & Threlfo (2002). 'EMDR in the treatment of chronic pain'. *Journal of Clinical Psychology* (online periodical), *58(12)*, 1505–1520.
3   See, among others: www.iasp-pain.org, 2020; Grant & Threlfo (2002); Verrier, P. (2003); Otis *et al.* (2003); Malchiodi, C., Ed. (1999).
4   Verrier, P. (2003). 'Docteur, ce n'est pas dans ma tête, j'ai vraiment mal'. *Le Médecin du Québec, 38(6)*, 53–60.
5   Beauchamp, P. (1995). 'Le soulagement de la douleur: aspect médical'. *Frontières* (online periodical), *8(2)*, 32–34. 33: Free translation.
6   Bourgault, P. Nursing professor, in *La Tribune* newspaper, Sherbrooke, November 21, 2006.
7   Association Québécoise de la Douleur Chronique. 'Composer avec la douleur chronique', published in the Quebec Press in November 2006.
8   According to Seyo *et al.* (1991), cited in Grant & Threlfo (2002). 'EMDR in the treatment of chronic pain.' *Journal of Clinical Psychology* (online periodical), *58(12)*, 1505–1520.
9   Weisberg *et al.* (1999), cited in Otis, J. D., Keane, T. M. & Kerns, R. D. (2003). 'An examination of the relationship between chronic pain and post-traumatic stress disorder'. *Journal of Rehabilitation Research and Development, 40(5)*, 397–406.
10  According to Otis, J. D.; Keane, T. M. & Kerns, R. D. (2003). 'An examination of the relationship between chronic pain and post-traumatic stress disorder'. *Journal of Rehabilitation Research and Development, 40(5)*, 397–406.

11 Beckham *et al.* (1997), cited in Otis, J. D.; Keane, T. M.; Kerns, R. D. (2003). 'An examination of the relationship between chronic pain and post-traumatic stress disorder'. *Journal of Rehabilitation Research and Development, 40(5)*, 397–406.

12 Bonin, M.; Norton, G. R.; Frombach, I. & Asmundson, G. J. G. (2000). 'PTSD in different treatment settings: a preliminary investigation of PTSD symptomatology in substance abuse and chronic pain patients'. *Depression and Anxiety, 11*, 131–133.

13 Verrier, P. (2003). 'Docteur, ce n'est pas dans ma tête, j'ai vraiment mal'. *Le Médecin du Québec, 38(6)*, 53–60.

14 Scaer, R. (2001). *The Body Bears the Burden, Trauma, Dissociation, and Disease.* Binghamton, NY: The Haworth Medical Press.

15 According to Solomon, S. (2005). 'Chronic post-traumatic neck and head pain'. *The Journal of Head & Face Pain* (online periodical), *45(1)*, 53–67.

16 See among others: Camic, (1999); Knight and Camic, (1998); Grant and Threlfo (2002) and Solomon, (2005).

17 Melzack, R.; Wall, P. D. (1965). 'Pain mechanisms: A new theory'. *Science 150*, 971–979, cited in Camic (1999). 'Expanding treatment possibilities for chronic pain through the expressive arts'. In: Malchiodi, C. Ed.). *Medical Art Therapy with Adults*, p. 46. Philadelphia, PA: Jessica Kingsley.

18 Camic, P. M. (1999). 'Expanding treatment possibilities for chronic pain through the expressive arts'. In: Malchiodi, C. Ed. (1999). *Medical Art Therapy with Adults*, 46. Philadelphia, PA: Jessica Kingsley.

19 Camic, P. M. *Op. Cit.* 47.

20 According to Otis J. D. *et al.* (2003).

# 3 Post-Traumatic Stress Disorder (PTSD)

*Johanne Hamel*

## Definition of post-traumatic stress disorder (PTSD)

Post-traumatic stress disorder (PTSD) is defined in the DSM-V Manual (2013) as follows:[1] Exposure to actual or threatened death, serious injury, or sexual violence in one or more of the following ways: the victim may have experience himself or herself the traumatic event, or may have witnessed in person the event as it occurred to others, or may have learned that a violent or accidental event has happened to a close family member or to a close friend. It may also be happening to first responders, police officers, or other persons who are repeatedly exposed to traumatic events (2013).

Four specific types of symptoms must be present for a diagnosis of PTSD to be made. There must be intrusion symptoms such as re-experiencing the trauma event, i.e. symptoms indicating that the traumatic event is constantly replayed, either by intrusive recollections, recurrent nightmares, or sudden impressions that the event is about to repeat itself or by very strong physiological or psychological distress responses when facing some internal or external cues recalling the event, even subtly.

There must also be a tendency to avoid trauma-associated thoughts, feelings, or conversations, as well as any activity, place or people recalling the trauma event. A blunting of the general reactivity, which is also a form of avoidance, can be noticed as well. This will typically manifest in the loss of interest or withdrawing from involvement in important activities, the feeling of becoming alien to others or being alienated from them, the inability to have tender feelings, or a sense of facing a dead end or a bleak future, as if life could not go on normally.

There will be negative alterations in cognitions and mood, such as the inability to remember an important aspect of a traumatic event, negative beliefs about oneself, persistent negative emotional state, diminished interest in life, or feeling estranged from others.

And finally, neuro-vegetative activation, as manifested, for example, in difficulty falling asleep or interrupted sleep, irritability or outbursts of anger, difficulty concentrating, hyper-vigilance (constant watch for danger), and exaggerated startle responses.

For a diagnostic of PTSD to be made, symptoms must last for more than one month and cause clinically significant distress or impairment of social, occupational, or other important life areas.

An acute stress response can also be diagnosed, which is characterized by symptoms similar to those of PTSD, including a state of dissociation.[2] Dissociation is the inability to recall important and usually traumatic personal memories, and this cannot be explained by bad memory alone. Sometimes, PTSD does not develop until three or even six months after a traumatic event.[3]

PTSD can develop as a result of traumatic events including exposure to violence (such as fighting in a war, bank robbery, terrorist acts, and sexual or physical abuse), a vehicle accident, a shipwreck, a fire, a medical procedure, a natural disaster (hurricane, tsunami, etc.) to name a few, or as a result of witnessing such incidents happening to others. However, not all victims or witnesses of such incidents will develop PTSD. Only about 25% to 35% of victims are likely to develop PTSD. Among the general population, 7% to 10% of people suffer from PTSD. It is worth noting that women are twice as likely as men to develop PTSD as a result of trauma.[4]

### *Usual treatments for PTSD*

The best known and current treatments for PTSD are the cognitive-behavioral approaches. To a lesser extent, eye movement desensitization and reprocessing (EMDR) is used successfully. Furthermore, according to Linda Chapman (2014), director of the Art Therapy Institute of the Redwoods in California, art therapy is widely used in hospitals in the USA based on its short-term effectiveness in treating trauma.

In the cognitive-behavioral approach, action is usually taken to counter-act the avoidance pattern that maintains or exacerbates PTSD symptoms; for this purpose, what constitutes PTSD is explained to the patient; intense emotions and ideas that bring shame, guilt, and distress and maintain the symptoms are worked on; the patients will be taught a relaxation method to manage their stress and gradual exposure *in vivo* or to the trauma memories are often suggested.[5] Other approaches focus on a more specific intervention on *dissociation*, which is considered as the causal factor of all the other symptoms.[6]

Among all these approaches, I have identified eight types of therapeutic goals that trauma therapists commonly pursue. They are the following: to facilitate abreaction (i.e. to help find and relive forgotten traumatic memories), to unfreeze the frozen motor reaction, to facilitate the expression of intense emotions related to trauma, to reduce the restricted affects, to reduce stress and promote relaxation, to create a safe haven, to rebuild personal identity, and finally, to regain personal integrity. Chapter 5 will address how art therapy can facilitate the achievement of each of these eight goals.

### Chronic pain in PTSD

First of all, it must be made clear that trauma and PTSD do not contribute to good physical health. Many studies report that many health problems go along with PTSD and that this disorder should be considered a negative factor in health.[7] The research demonstrated that even after having controlled for a large number of factors affecting health, PTSD remains a negative intermediate for health.[8] Chronic pain is one of the common health problems associated with PTSD. Indeed, it is becoming increasingly clear that a background of physical or sexual abuse or any other trauma is a risk factor for somatization and painful disorders such as fibromyalgia, pelvic pain, irritable bowel syndrome, etc.[9]

Clinical practice and research suggest that chronic pain and PTSD show high comorbidity and could even interact in ways that negatively influence the course of one or the other; however, there has been relatively limited research on the matter to date.[10]

Asmundson, Coons, Taylor & Katz (2002) also found that chronic pain and PTSD are commonly comorbid and believe that they maintain each other through common mechanisms, such as fear and avoidance, anxiety sensitivity, and a tendency to catastrophizing. In addition, it seems that the presence of both increases the severity of the symptoms of both conditions.[11]

Given the common comorbidity of these two conditions, recommendations are as follows:

- Clinicians seeing patients with PTSD symptoms should also assess the presence of chronic pain such as fibromyalgia or chronic musculoskeletal pain; and
- Conversely, patients complaining of pain, especially chronic pain, should also be assessed for the presence of PTSD.[12]

Asmundson, Wright, McCreary, and Pedlar[13] also suggest that PTSD symptoms such as physiological response to triggers, restricted affects, the feeling of facing a dead end, and hyper-vigilance could become more prominent when there is also chronic pain. They believe that chronic pain most likely exerts its influence by increasing hyper-vigilance: sufferers pay attention to anything that could increase their pain. In a study comparing a group with chronic pain with a non-suffering group of veterans, this pattern was obvious, but not statistically significant. Further research is needed to determine the specific mechanisms that explain this cumulative impact of pain on PTSD.

Other researchers[14] have also found that higher levels of re-experiencing symptoms are associated with higher levels of pain and disability related to pain, and that patients with chronic pain related to trauma or PTSD experience more intense pain and emotional distress, higher levels of disruption in life, as well as greater disability than patients with pain, without trauma, or PTSD.

I tend to view pain as a sort of somatic re-experiencing of a traumatic event (flashback). The most known re-experiencing occurrences are visual or auditory, but although we are less familiar with them, Rothschild[15] postulates that emotional, behavioural, or somatic flashbacks can also occur, based on Levine's SIBAM (sensation, image, behavior, affect, and meaning) model (See chapter 7). She states that:

Instances of hyper-arousal, hyper-startle reflex, otherwise unexplainable emotional upset, physical pain, or intense irritation can all be easily explained by the phenomenon of flashback (2000, p. 70).

Otis *et al.* (2003) identify three models in particular to explain the relationship between chronic pain and PTSD. Even if the authors consider that these models are not sufficiently tested empirically, it is interesting to look into them. They are the following:[16]

Sharp and Harvey's (2001) mutual maintenance model proposes seven specific maintenance factors:

1   Attention bias may be present in chronic pain and PTSD patients, such that they attend to threatening or painful stimuli;
2   Anxiety sensitivity may contribute toward a vulnerability to catastrophize;
3   Pain can be a reminder of the traumatic event, triggering an arousal response, avoidance of the cause of pain, and of any memories of the trauma;
4   In both disorders, avoidance can be adopted as a means to minimize pain and disturbing thoughts;
5   Fatigue and lethargy associated with depression can contribute to both disorders;
6   General anxiety can contribute to both disorders;
7   Cognitive demands from symptoms of pain and PTSD limit the use of adaptive coping strategies.

The second model is the shared vulnerability hypothesis of Asmundson *et al.* (2002), in which anxiety sensitivity would be a predisposing factor for the development of both conditions.

The third model is the modified fear-avoidance model of Norton and Asmundson (2003), which emphasizes the contributions of physiological symptoms and overactivation, such as increased blood flow, heart rate, or muscle tension, which could directly increase sensations of pain and reinforce fears and negative beliefs that physical activity is trying. Patients would interpret these physical sensations as being related to pain.

### Treatment of chronic pain associated with PTSD

The purpose here is to review the existing treatments when both chronic pain and trauma are present and to verify their effectiveness. Presenting these methods will help to understand the principles on the basis of which they work, principles that also underlie the art therapy interventions outlined in Part 4, chapter 10.

After reviewing the existing research on the treatment of PTSD with coexisting chronic pain, previously mentioned authors (Otis *et al.* (2000) concluded the following:

- Standard cognitive-behavioral methods such as cognitive restructuring, training in day-to-day management skills and relaxation, psycho-education on the avoidance mechanism, exposure activities and exposure to interoceptive sensations to cope with uncomfortable physiological sensations, are all helpful methods
- Other interventions could also be helpful, such as the ones on confidence in self-efficacy, remediation of attention biases and reduction of catastrophic expectations
- There are few studies on the matter, and more research is needed to develop effective treatments

Other authors,[17] however, recommend that the cognitive-behavioral strategies for treating PTSD be adapted to include pain management strategies. They also suggest integrating treatments to reduce anxiety sensitivity, which would alleviate the symptoms of both PTSD and chronic pain. According to them, the most powerful method would be the interoceptive exposure therapy, i.e. exposure to internal sensations instead of their avoidance, which is actually a key principle in somatic art therapy.

There is no systematic empirical research indicating that the treatment would be more effective by addressing one of the conditions first (PTSD or chronic pain) instead of treating them simultaneously.[18]

Sometimes the pain decreases simply by treating PTSD. A case study[19] shows that treating the cause of pain (meaning PTSD) can be effective in relieving pain. They report the case of a 36-year-old woman who went to a pain management clinic for an unexplained hand pain and numbness symptoms. Having experienced trauma as a teenager, she was diagnosed with a conversion reaction and PTSD. After a successful exposure-based therapy, her physical symptoms, perceived as well as objectively measured, decreased dramatically.

However, few specific treatments for pain sensation appear to exist as related to PTSD work. I found three examples of trauma treatments used specifically for pain: somatic experiencing (SE), EMDR and hypnosis. Only the EMDR approach has received some scientific validation to date.

### Scaer and Levine's Somatic Experiencing approach[20]

Robert Scaer (2001) worked predominantly with motor vehicle accident victims who subsequently developed PTSD. He successfully used Levine's

Somatic Experiencing (SE) (1997) to treat chronic pain. While he acknowledged that SE received little scientific validation, he was also very impressed with its efficacy in the treatment of chronic pain and myofascial pain, among others. The myofascial type of pain is recognizable by some sensitive muscular zones with very specific painful points. Myofascial pain is ubiquitous in the chronic pain population and extremely resistant to treatment.[21]

His positive results are based on his experience with several hundred patients treated with both SE or with EMDR (see next page for an explanation on this method). His conclusion is that SE tends to result in resolution of dissociative traits and behaviors more effectively than many other techniques.[22] Now the relation between dissociation and the maintenance of PTSD symptoms will be addressed in more detail in chapter 7.

Scaer and Levine use the felt sense to pursue and access the trauma response. According to Scaer, the felt sense is the sum total of all sensations from all sense organs, both conscious and subliminal, at any given moment.[23] The felt sense becomes accessible if one concentrates purposely on feeling the subtleties of somatic awareness just as in somatic art therapy.

SE involves exploration of these sensations by the patient under the guidance of a therapist trained in the technique. Here is how Scaer describes the process, using the concept of somasthetic procedural memory, which is basically the recollection of all movements made or not made (frozen) to protect oneself during the traumatic event:

'When patients with PTSD or its late manifestations access the felt sense, they will eventually arrive at awareness of subtle somatic sensations that represent somasthetic procedural memory for a traumatic experience. The patients will then be guided initially to experience the sensation more intensely, and then to retreat to a previously established imaginary "safe place" as they begin to experience arousal triggered by the developing link to the limbic portion of that memory. By titrating in and out of this "trauma vortex" with the guidance of the therapist, the patient will eventually undergo the stereotyped motor and autonomic "discharge" of traumatic energy typified in animals emerging from the freeze response. (…) It will usually involve an involuntary motor response that often reflects the movement patterns experienced in a protective fashion during the traumatic event. "Completion" of that movement is felt to be an important event in dissipation of the procedural memory for the trauma and its link to arousal.'

(Scaer, 2001, p. 170)

### *Eye movement desensitization and reprocessing*

Grant and Threlfo (2002) used eye movement desensitization and reprocessing (EMDR) to treat three patients suffering with chronic pain for at least six months and showing feelings of emotional distress; the treatment lasted nine weeks with weekly one-hour sessions. Only one patient had previously experienced a trauma (a motorcycle accident). The three patients noticed substantial decreases in pain following treatment, and these changes lasted for at least two months (two years at least for one patient; the two others could not be reached for a follow-up after two years). The three patients also noticed a decrease in emotional distress, including a decreased tendency to catastrophic expectations. The traumatized person also reported that her symptoms decreased.[24]

These findings have virtually no generalizability, given that there were only three patients. They are certainly of interest for more systematic research. The hypotheses about the effectiveness of EMDR in this research also appear of great interest, mainly because of the inclusion of emotional therapy. Indeed, the authors believe that desensitizing the emotional aspects of the pain could be the factor operating in EMDR, this hypothesis being consistent with research about the involvement of the limbic system in nociception.[25] According to them, EMDR could allow the separation of the connections between traumatic memories and painful associations, which allows less distressful replays of the memories and concomitant changes in behavior.

For them, trauma treatment with EMDR, which focuses on the emotional, somatic, and cognitive aspects, allows for more consistent changes and offer advantages over more conventional approaches that fail to take into account the emotional side of pain.

### Hypnosis

Muraoka, Komiyama, Hosoi, Mine, and Kubo (1996) used hypnosis successfully to treat phantom limb pain with PTSD. Antidepressant drugs were used as well. In 1945, at the age of 16, the patient had witnessed his parents' death during the atomic bomb explosion in Hiroshima. At the age of 31, he also had suffered critical injuries in a train crash, and his left leg had to be amputated without anesthesia after having been nearly severed.

Working with cognitive restructuring through hypnosis, the authors first asked the patient to imagine his left leg as healthy and whole as the right leg, and they were able to achieve results after three months: severe pain was occurring only intermittently, and oral pain medication was significantly decreased.

They achieved even better results by asking the patient to visualize under hypnosis that his leg was gradually decreasing in size. After one year, the patient started noticing that the phantom limb sensations ceased for several hours a day, and pain had significantly decreased. While the authors are aware that hypnosis is often not considered a viable treatment method, they argue that any conventional form of treatment alone proves insufficient to alleviate the pain in cases of very intense trauma and suggest further investigation on this method.

# Notes

1 See Appendix A for an excerpt from the DSM-V (2013) about PTSD.
2 American Psychiatric Association. (2013). Op. Cit.
3 American Psychiatric Association. (2013). Op. Cit.
4 For more information on these data, please see Brillon, P. (2017). Comment aider les victimes souffrant de stress post-traumatique. Guide à l'intention des thérapeutes. Montréal, Qc.: Québec-Livres.
5 See Brillon, P. (2017). *Comment aider les victimes souffrant de stress post-traumatique. Guide à l'intention des thérapeutes.* Montréal, Qc.: Québec-Livres.
6 See among others Levine, P. (1997), Van der Kolk, B. (1994) and Scaer, R. (2001). These authors will be discussed in Chapter 7.
7 See Schnurr, P. P. (1996). 'Trauma, PTSD, and physical health'. *The National Center for Post-Traumatic Stress Disorder Research Quarterly, 7(3)*, as well as Friedman, M. J. & Schnurr, P. P. (1996). 'Trauma, PTSD, and Health.' *NCP Clinical Quarterly* (online periodical), *6(4)*.
8 Lauterbach, D., Vora, R. & Rakow, M. (2005). 'The relationship between posttraumatic stress disorder and self-reported health problems'. *Psychosomatic Medicine* (online periodical), *67(6)*, 939–947.
9 Verrier, P. (2003). 'Docteur, ce n'est pas dans ma tête, j'ai vraiment mal'. *Le Médecin du Québec, 38(6)*, 53–60.
10 Otis, J. D.; Keane, T. M. & Kerns, R. D. (2003). 'An examination of the relationship between chronic pain and post-traumatic stress disorder'. *Journal of Rehabilitation Research and Development, 40(5)*.
11 Otis *et al.* (2003): *Op. Cit.*
12 According to Asmundson, G. J. G., Coons, M. J., Taylor, S. & Katz, J. (2002). 'PTSD and the experience of pain: research and clinical implications of shared vulnerability and mutual maintenance models'. *Canadian Journal of Psychiatry, 47(10)*, 930–937.
13 Asmundson, G. J. G., Wright, K. D., McCreary, D. R. & Pedlar, D. (2003). 'Post-traumatic stress disorder symptoms in United Nations peacekeepers with and without chronic pain'. *Cognitive Behavior Therapy, 32(1)*, 26–37.
14 Otis, J. D., Keane, T. M. & Kerns, R. D. (2003). 'An examination of the relationship between chronic pain and post-traumatic stress disorder'. *Journal of Rehabilitation Research and Development, 40(5)*, 397–406.
15 Rothschild, B. (2000). *The Body Remembers. The Psychophysiology of Trauma and Trauma Treatment.* New York, NY: W. W. Norton & Co.
16 Otis *et al.* (2003), *Op. Cit.*, p. 400.
17 Asmundson, G. J. G., Coons, M. J., Taylor, S. & Katz, J. (2002). 'PTSD and the experience of pain: research and clinical implications of shared vulnerability and mutual maintenance models'. *Canadian Journal of Psychiatry, 47(10)*, 930–937.
18 According to Asmundson, G. J. G., Wright, K. D., McCreary, D. R. & Pedlar, D. (2003). 'Post-traumatic stress disorder symptoms in United Nations peacekeepers with and without chronic pain'. *Cognitive Behavior Therapy, 32(1)*, 26–37.
19 Ciano-Federoff, L. M. & Sperry, J. A. (2005) are the authors of this case study. 'On "Converting" hand pain into psychological pain: treating hand pain vicariously through exposure-based therapy for PTSD'. *Clinical Case Studies, 4(1)*, 57–71.
20 The Somatic Experiencing approach, developed by P. Levine, 1997.
21 Scaer, R. (2001). *The Body Bears the Burden. Trauma, Dissociation, and Disease.* Binghamton, NY: The Haworth Medical Press.

22 Scaer, R. (2001). *Op. Cit.*
23 Scaer, R. (2001). *Op. Cit.*
24 Grant, M. & Threlfo, C. (2002). 'EMDR in the treatment of chronic pain'. *Journal of Clinical Psychology* (online periodical), *58(12)*.
25 Grant, M. & Threlfo, C. (2002), *Op. Cit.*

# Part II

# An Overview of Art Therapy Treatments

# 4 Art Therapy for PTSD and Chronic Pain

## An Overview

*Johanne Hamel*

The chapter reviews art therapeutic treatments for chronic pain, as well as the existing specialized documentation about art therapist's adult clients suffering from post-traumatic stress disorder (PTSD). Three special art therapy protocols for PTSD treatment are outlined.

## Art therapy treatments for chronic pain: Examples

To my knowledge, no writing exists on the treatment of chronic pain through art therapy with regard to PTSD. However, I found three examples of therapeutic work specifically related to pain: one for groups, and the other two for individual sessions.

### Group therapy on chronic pain through creative arts

Camic (1999) wrote about the use of expressive arts to treat chronic pain. In a pain management group, he used visual arts (drawing, painting, sculpture, collage), writing (poetry, narrative writing, diary), music, meditation, and guided imagery. Although he does not use only art therapy, his study is included here because it is one of the very few on chronic pain.

Like many others, he considers that strategies for pain management rather than for pain healing are more appropriate, which is basically what he proposed for a group experience that was conducted over 15 weeks, with weekly sessions of 90 minutes.[1] He worked with seven men suffering with mild chronic pain.

He believes that expressive arts should be integrated to chronic pain management because the cognitive-behavioral approach fails to help all chronic pain sufferers.[2] He uses visual arts to achieve the following goals:

- To help patients to keep their mind off the pain;
- To help them to make sense of their pain;
- To help them to relax;
- To help them to mourn the loss of their physical functioning.

In a very touching testimonial, he told how he was able to help his father, who was suffering from cancer at the time that he was writing a chapter of his book about pain. He and his father spent several hours working on art projects, whereas before, his father was dying in bed. His use of drawing, painting, 1919 photographs, old newspaper articles, and letters for a collage allowed his father to make sense of his final days while diverting his attention from that.[3]

Distractions seem to have a valid therapeutic purpose, as demonstrated by Solomon's study (2005)[4], which indicates that waiting and paying attention to pain can prolong and amplify pain while stopping to wait and distractions can have the opposite effect. Camic regrets that there is limited research proving the value and importance of integrating creative arts approaches, such as art therapy in the treatment of chronic pain.

### Multiple personality disorder and acute pain

Treating a patient suffering from multiple personality disorder (MPD), Jacobson (1994) used art therapy to work on acute pain. She tells about a client who developed pain in her buttock muscles after several months of art therapy, without any medical cause. Through the use of collage, finger painting (at the request of one of her sub-personalities), and two drawings, a traumatic memory came back and was worked on in several partial abreaction sessions, followed by a complete one. Following this series of four art creations and the recollection of repeated anal rapes by his father, the body memories and pain of her client were resolved.[5] It should be noted that this brief therapy work must be understood in the context of a longstanding pre-existing therapeutic relationship.

Jacobson developed a special procedure for working with patients with MPD. This procedure is called 'stepping in'. As an example, she asked one of the dissociated sub-personalities of a client to 'try the body on the table', drawn by another sub-personality, and to take a few seconds to check whether or not this experience could also correspond to hers. The client had been gang-raped by four adult men, including her father. The author considers that the 'stepping in' method enables the sharing of the dissociated material between the sub-personalities within the entire system, which reduces the need for dissociation and supports the reintegration of the psyche.[6]

### Sandplay therapy and medical trauma

Finally, let's mention the case of a five-year-old boy attending Sandplay therapy sessions for serious physical problems. Josh had gone through years of medical trauma and was absolutely unwilling to defecate. His process was facilitated by playing. He began throwing large amounts of sand up in the air and repeated this several times while having a lot of flatulence. He started going to the bathroom in the same week. His immune system subsequently strengthened, and he was able to fight the disease. After a few months, he was strong enough to undergo a medical procedure, and his disease was cured.[7] I am mentioning it here because, although it would certainly be different in an adult, it is noteworthy that Sandplay therapy can help out with physiology. Moreover, it is likely that it could be used with adults for that purpose, as mentioned by Carey (2006). [8]

## Art therapy and PTSD

While art therapy is a very common treatment for PTSD in the USA, there are relatively few articles on the matter in specialized journals, and only a few books address the treatment of trauma through art therapy.[9] As for chronic pain, research is virtually non-existent.

With rare exceptions, we will not address research into art therapy with children suffering from PTSD nor articles dealing with art therapy in conjunction with other types of creative arts like music, poetry, performing arts, etc. However, it is interesting to note that other creative arts often serve to treat PTSD, especially music and performing arts.[10] The subject of this book is restricted to adults suffering from PTSD or trauma in general and from chronic pain.

Art therapists work with a broad range of medicalized or traumatized clients. The documented interventions do not refer only to persons officially diagnosed with PTSD. As for medical art therapy, I found professional art therapists working with people who had a stroke, underwent laryngectomy procedures, or mastectomy procedures; and those suffering from AIDS, cancer, tuberculosis, or people with disabilities.[11] Their research can prove to be relevant, given the health problems that PTSD sufferers usually have.

Among the traumatized clients, we find interventions with burn victims[12] and veterans.[13] Other professionals work with persons suffering from a dissociative identity disorder (DID) or MPD.[14] As these last syndromes have been clearly linked to severe and repeated childhood abuse,[15] this type of research is directly related to the topic covered herein. Jacobson (1994) in particular addresses abreaction, which she defines as 'the process of becoming aware of previously unconscious material or recalling and re-experiencing such material'.[16] She demonstrates how art therapy facilitates the recollection of trauma memories and helps to embrace abreaction.

### *Sexual abuse*

However, the most documented trauma in art therapy is definitely sexual abuse. Two French-Canadian psychologists and art therapists, Lambert and Simard (1997), explain how they use art therapy with female victims of sexual abuse during childhood and adolescence. Many American authors also reported art therapeutic interventions with these clients.[17]

Interventions are varied and have a number of different goals: to promote the expression of emotions related to past traumatic experiences; to facilitate and support the building of self-esteem; to reduce stress and to take legal or family actions should the patient want to do so.[18]

### Collective disasters

A number of art therapy interventions were also conducted with groups of survivors of collective disasters. Jones (1997) worked for six months with survivors of the terrorist destruction of the Oklahoma City Federal Building in April 1995. The interventions included emotional maps and bridging exercises, as well as exercises to express specific feelings such as guilt, anger, and grief, to help to resolve grief and loss, as well as to build self-esteem and self-confidence. After one year, all art therapy group participants returned to work and continued to progress, which was not necessarily true for participants in other groups. Along the same lines,[19] some worked with young teenagers to create a mural after the 9/11 events.

### Immigrant women and inmates

Other therapists[20] worked with immigrant women using Sandplay therapy, while others used drawings, collages, and three-dimensional construction forms. All of them were physically and sexually abused.

Creating a safe place for them, another art therapist[21] worked with female inmates with a history of severe trauma, for the purpose of allowing them to reconnect with unstated thoughts, feelings, and fantasies and to express their feelings appropriately.

This shows that art therapists are working actively to treat trauma with various clients suffering from a range of problems, as much in individual sessions as in groups, in multiple contexts.

Bessel van der Kolk[22], whose work will be discussed in more detail in chapter 7, used artwork with a 30-year-old woman referred for serious insecurity problems, compulsive behaviors, and unusual somatic symptoms; she was diagnosed with PTSD. She had a history of multiple sexual traumas. After painting her dreams, she analysed them as well as her drawings. She was able to gradually recollect trauma memories and integrate them.

After 13 months, her therapy was less about trauma (although she still had partial amnesia) and more about the 'here and now' and future prospects. She was considering a pregnancy and questioning her career path. Van der Kolk believes that the 'painting cure' can be used to recollect and integrate traumatic memories with talented individuals (what he calls special cognitive resources), but does not go as far as extending the use of art to other types of trauma victims.

**Art therapy protocols for PTSD treatments**

Some specific protocols for PTSD treatment have been developed over the past 15 years. Gantt and Tinnin (2009) developed mayor guidelines for trauma therapy based on the instinctual trauma response (ITR). They propose a whole sequence of drawings and actions for clients to go through. The ITR is a universal reaction to trauma, an instinctual survival strategy, made up of six different survival responses. They describe the ITR this way (2009):

In the throes of trauma, a human tries first to execute intentional action. If that fails, consciousness yields to reflexive mammalian flight or fight; if that fails, the person responds with the reptilian freeze. In effect, higher cortical functions go 'offline', as it were (p. 149).

Other survival strategies resulting from the freeze response, include numbing and loss of proprioception, feeling of loss of all connection to the body (depersonalization) or an out-of-body experience bringing an altered state of consciousness and distortion of perception. Coming out of the freeze stage, the person might adopt a submissive behavior and will eventually adopt self-repair strategies, healthy or not (drugs, alcohol, etc.).

They suggest a series of drawings to restore better functioning, aiming first and foremost at making the event become past tense instead of the client experiencing the trauma as if it was still happening and feeling stuck in the experience. I have seen clients use this protocol successfully.

In their *Graphic Narrative Processing*, the client goes through the following steps:

- The therapist explains the phases of the instinctual trauma response (ITR) to the client
- The therapist instructs the client to create a narrative of the trauma story in pictures, always including the self as viewed from the emotionally detached perspective of an observer
- The client creates before and after pictures
- The client labels each picture with the appropriate phase of the ITR such as: startle response, flight/fight, freeze, altered state of consciousness (out-of-body experience), submission or self-repair
- The client displays the complete narrative for everyone to see
- The client becomes the audience as the therapist tells the story depicted by the pictures
- Afterwards they suggest that the client might do a dialogue with the frozen part of self, speaking, drawing, or writing for each part in turn

Hass-Cohen and Clyde Findlay (2019) propose a protocol of four drawings based on relational neuroscience and memory reconsolidation, called ATRN-MR. It is designed to 'visually and vividly compete with the old memories' (p. 57) to facilitate a memory reconsolidation (MR). It can be done in one or two sessions.

The activation of a traumatic memory may give rise to the building of a new way of perceiving the event and oneself, thus a memory reconsolidation. The traumatic recalling must be brief, no more than an hour, and allow for new information to come into the story. The sequence of four drawings is as follows:

- In the first drawing, the person is asked to draw a picture of the problem. It is best to spend little time in this drawing and have a low arousal level to avoid re-traumatizing the client
- In the second drawing, the person is asked to draw a self-portrait. It shows typically the debilitating effect of the event on the self-image of the client
- In the third drawing, the client is asked to draw the external and internal resources that helped her or him in the past and in the present. The pleasure of creativity and of recalling positive resources.... 'may help mitigate the strength of the trauma reminder (the first drawing) and reduce emotive arousal, cognitive distortions and re-traumatizing' (p. 57)
- The last drawing, a self-portrait of how the client sees herself or himself now, is looked at in full view of the resources picture, which encourages a new self-perspective

The whole protocol will likely help mitigate or eliminate negative impacts of the trauma on day-to-day functioning.

Finally, Talwar (2007) designed an art therapy trauma protocol (ATTP) to access traumatic somatic memories and reduce their impact. The ATTP protocol involves drawing or painting in a standing position, using alternatively the right and left hands. After verbally processing the traumatic event, the client is asked to draw the somatic residual memory of the event, as well as her or his negative self-perception followed by the desired positive self-perception. They do so .... 'until there are no longer any feelings of disturbance on the recall of the traumatic event' (p. 31). This technique focuses exclusively on processing somatic memory. It helps emotional processing and left-brain/right brain integration by switching between dominant and non-dominant hands, changing sheets of paper every time. Talwar's clients reported positive results. This technique might not be pertinent for every client, as some ego-strength is necessary before processing the trauma.

There are many considerations in applying these protocols, and I strongly suggest art therapists to read and study these authors' writings before using these powerful treatment protocols.

## Notes

1 Camic, P. *Op. Cit.*, 47–48.
2 Camic, P. *Op. Cit.*, 47–48.
3 Camic, P. *Op. Cit.*, 47–48.

4 Solomon, S. (2005). *Op. Cit.*
5 Jacobson, M. (1994). *Op. Cit.*
6 Jacobson, M. (1994). *Op. Cit.*
7 McCarthy, D. in: Carey, L. (2006). *Expressive and Creative Arts Methods for Trauma Survivors.* London and Philadelphia, PA: Jessica Kingsley.
8 Carey, L. (2006): *Op. Cit.*
9 See Malchiodi (2020), Carey, (Ed.), 2006; Malchiodi, 1999; Spencer, 1997 as well as Cohen, Barnes & Rankin, 1995.
10 See Camic, P. M. (1999). *Op. Cit.*
11 See Malchiodi, C. (1999). *Op. Cit.*
12 Russel, J. (1995). 'Art therapy on a hospital burn unit: A step towards healing and recovery'. *Art Therapy, Journal of the American Art Therapy Association, 12(1),* 39–45.
13 Golub, D., 1985; Greece, M., 2003; Johnson, D. R., 1987; Berkowitz, S., 1990 as well as Hines-Martin, V. P. & Ising, M., 1993.
14 Engle, P. (1997). Art therapy and dissociative disorders'. *Art Therapy, Journal of the American Art Therapy Association, 14*(4), 246–254, as well as Jacobson, M. (1994). 'Abreacting and assimilating traumatic, dissociated memories of MPD patients through art therapy.' *Art Therapy, Journal of the American Art Therapy Association, 11(1),* 48–52.
15 See Kluft, R. P. (1984), cited in Jacobson, M. (1994). *Op. Cit.*
16 Jacobson, M. (1994), p. 48. *Op. Cit.*
17 Among them, Anderson (1995); Lev-Wiesel (1998); Landgarten (1990); Howard (1990); Brooke (1995); Estep, (1995); Hargrave-Nykaza (1994); Waller (1992) and Powel & Faherty (1990).
18 Lambert, J. & Simard, P. (1997). 'L'art-thérapie, approche auprès des femmes adultes victimes d'agression à caractère sexuel durant l'enfance ou l'adolescence'. *Revue Québécoise de Psychologie, 18(3),* 203–228.
19 Mapp, I. & Koch, D. (2004). Creation of a group mural to promote healing following a mass trauma, in: Webb, N. B. (Ed.). *Mass Trauma and Violence: Helping Families and Children Cope.* New York, NY: Guilford.
20 Lacroix, L. (2002). 'Retour au pays d'origine. Créativité sensorielle par l'utilisation du jeu de sable en art-thérapie'. *Prisme,* 37 (Online periodical), as well as Heusch, N. & Shermarke, M. (2001). 'Art-thérapie et reconstruction identitaire: Dévoilement d'expériences traumatiques dans un groupe de femmes réfugiées'. *Prisme,* 35.
21 Merriam, B. (1998). 'To find a voice: art therapy in a woman's prison', *Women and Therapy, 21(1),* 157–171.
22 Van der Kolk, B. A. (1987). *Psychological Trauma.* Washington, DC: American Psychiatric Press.

# 5 Trauma Treatment
## Eight Techniques for Art Therapists

*Johanne Hamel*

In reviewing other approaches commonly used to treat trauma, including the cognitive-behavioral approach (Brillon, 2017a, 2017b) the author found many techniques in the art therapy specialized documentation that actually pursue the same goals than those other approaches and are useful to treat trauma. This chapter surveys these art therapeutic techniques, all approaches combined. Indeed, beyond particular approaches and different theoretical rationales, psychoanalyst, humanistic, or others, a know-how specific to the discipline of art therapy is gradually developing, with more and more common and proven methods of intervention. These art therapy techniques apply equally to trauma victims with or without a PTSD diagnosis. Research indicates that chronic pain and post-traumatic stress disorder (PTSD) symptoms need to be managed simultaneously to treat pain effectively.[1] The techniques presented in this chapter have been grouped into eight types, depending on what therapeutic purpose they address in terms of treating PTSD:

- Abreaction techniques
- Motor reaction de-freezing techniques
- Intense emotional expression techniques
- Affect restoration techniques
- Stress reduction and relaxation techniques
- Safe haven techniques
- Identity reconstruction techniques
- Personal integrity restoration techniques

## Abreaction techniques

Just about any art therapy technique will readily reveal the presence of trauma if a safe therapeutic relationship is established. Jacobson,[2] who works with patients suffering from the multiple personality disorder (MPD), also sees it that way:

In working with patients diagnosed with MPD, the invitation to draw or sculpt typically leads to the presentation of personal nightmares related to previous abuse.[3]

In my clinical experience, I observed the same with traumatized clients. Jacobson uses collage, spontaneous drawing, and her 'stepping in' technique.[4] The spontaneous drawing technique is quite appropriate to help recollection and facilitate the emotional abreaction that often occurs with it. Art therapists simply ask the clients to let their hand draw what comes spontaneously, with the medium of their choice. If instructions are given, they will be very open: 'Just let your drawings reflect how you feel right now', for example.

## Motor reaction de-freezing techniques

As we will see in chapter 7, according to Levine's[5] theory and clinical experience, de-freezing the motor reaction can prove tremendously useful in trauma treatment. De-freezing can be precisely enabled by a number of art therapy techniques, especially Sandplay[6] and puppetry interventions.[7] For example, patients can symbolically re-enact the trauma events with puppets and imagine while playing that their aggressors can cause no more harm, through effectively engaging their ability to defend themselves. This technique can be used with children as well as adults.[8]

## Intense emotional expression techniques

### Clay and 3-dimentional media

The use of clay, which can be beaten, throttled, and crushed, and of other three-dimensional media, for the expression of one's feelings of rage and aggressive instinct, allows the expression and regulation of intense affects in a safe environment. Pounding on a piece of wood with nails and a hammer might be very effective. Throwing tempera on a large paper is also useful, as long as the paint stays on the paper and does not get thrown on themselves, the wall or the therapist. Therapeutically, any intensity of emotion is acceptable, but aggressive behaviors are not. It helps to explain to clients that we do not have control over our emotions, that we can only accept them or repress them, but we need to control our behaviors when angry, which is much easier if the anger is conscious and accepted.

### The red lines exercise

Using a dry medium, it involves drawing with oil pastels red lines (anger) or black lines (rage) from the bottom of the sheet and pointing upward (symbolizing another specific person outside), but never towards the client. Oil pastels can be strongly pushed on the paper and that is why they are especially useful. I ask the client to repeat the lines on many papers, talking at the same time to the persons with whom the client is angry, expressing anger, one person at a time. Reluctance to express anger fully can be seen in the lines being weak, not really 'angry', going towards the sides of the paper instead of directly ahead, or in a soft tone of voice or polite words. I might encourage the client to express fully, giving examples with a few well-chosen insults! Polite and controlled 'I' messages are not helpful here! I explain that anger not fully expressed might come out in hurtful ways and that we have better control on our behavior if we can first fully express the feelings in a safe and contained way on paper. Then, afterwards, in real life, this energy can be used to assert oneself in a healthy way. Anger is how we know our emotional limits and what is not acceptable to us.

With this exercise, the experience is modulated in intensity, because clients' reluctance to express their anger is respected, explored, and gradually transcended. Meaningful work is done through clarifying moral objections or fears about expressing anger and through understanding that repressed anger turns into depression or physical pain. It might take a few sessions for a client to be able to express anger fully, and we might have to come back to it many times before it is accepted.

Another way that the reluctance might come out is by the clients saying that they are angry towards themselves. This is retroflected anger directed toward the self to avoid being angry. Saying 'Other than yourself, who are you angry with?' is a good way to bypass retroflection. If the client insists on drawing the lines from top to bottom towards themselves, I then ask what these lines might be saying if they could talk. They will immediately hear the retroflection, blaming themselves or diminishing their own value for instance. That helps clients accept directing the lines toward the person with whom they are really angry.[9]

Finally, Jobin (2002) proposes three exercises for working on emotional wounds that could prove useful for facilitating emotional expression:

My wound:

What does my wound look like? Is it a broken heart, an open wound, a fallen tree? Drawing spontaneously, use colours and shapes in an attempt to highlight your emotional wound. Then initiate a dialogue with it. When did it occur? What is needed? Write quickly, without restrictions.

The wounded child:

With your non-dominant hand, draw the wounded child inside you. Then, initiate a dialogue with her/him, using your usual hand for the voice of the adult and the other hand for the child. Ask her/him how she/he feels, what she/he needs, what you can do to help her/him heal, etc. Make sure to give her/him what she/he is asking for during the week or do the exercise called 'healing space' (see p. 36 of this book).

Releasing what is in your heart; nurturing the heart:

This is a two-step exercise using two pages. First, let's get it off your chest. What emotions, thoughts and sensations related to your wound have always been with you and poison your life? Use writing or drawing to release what is in your heart, avoid censoring yourself, and include everything. Then use the second page and ask yourself what nurtures your heart, makes you feel good and soothes you. What could you do to protect yourself, feel nurtured and heal? Make a list and illustrate this if you like. Circle one or two actions to be taken this week (2002, p. 188–190) (Free translation).

In art therapy sessions, grieving, mourning, pleasure and any other emotions are easily expressed on paper, which is facilitated by the art therapist suggesting specific art media suitable for the psychodynamics that are present (felt pen, pastels, finger paint, etc.).

## Affect restoration techniques

Restricted affects often occur as a result of trauma. Out of touch with their emotions, their physical sensations and their memories, the traumatized persons might no longer understand their intense reactions. Art allows the person undergoing therapy to reclaim everything that they are out of touch with, in a gentle and gradual way. By adapting to their pace and respecting their reluctance, the art therapist enables a safe and progressive journey. Often, the dam will suddenly give way when the person is ready.

Duchastel (2005, 178–180) provides a very interesting example, about 'Madeline':

When I ask Madeline, a 60-year-old, how she feels, it is like I am speaking a foreign language. Looking at me with a puzzled expression, she replies that she does not know. I invite her to close her eyes and focus on her breathing, then on her body sensations at this moment. She suddenly opens her eyes, looking panicked, and says 'I do not feel anything'. (....)

When she shares traumatic events in her life, she does it in a neutral manner similar to a news reader. Anyone who has experienced the same deeply hurtful situations would normally feel pain, anger, and/or distress. But Madeline feels nothing special. She does not acknowledge her emotions, she protects herself from them. However, the sudden onset of large red patches indicates that her body is in great trouble. As she rebels every time that I remark that an emotion is expressed in her body, I soon stopped pointing it out to her.

One day when she was sharing one of these hurtful events, a small teardrop-shaped red spot took shape under her right eye. It made her look very saddened even though at the tone of her voice, we would have sworn that everything was fine. Pretending to ignore this treacherous redness, I invited her to make her self-portrait in front of a mirror. She had been working for a long time, totally absorbed in it, when she suddenly turned to me with tears in her eyes: She just said 'I actually feel sad, so very sad about what happened', while wiping the tears running down her cheeks (2005, 178–180). (Free translation).

## Stress reduction and relaxation techniques

Jobin (2002, 174–176) proposes three techniques to work on stress and calm down:

My stress:

Draw your stress spontaneously. What does it look like? Does it feel like a knot in your guts, is it like a pit in the stomach, a lump in the throat, a ball of tangled wool? Doing it spontaneously, use colors and shapes that make sense to you, then write all the words that come to mind, around the edge of the drawing. Next, write down your thoughts about it.

Mr. Tense, Mrs. Uptight:

Imagine that your stress is a character. It rules your life and whispers in your ear 'You should do this and you should do that, You will never make it', etc. What does this character look like? What is it saying to you? What is its name? Make a drawing of it and around the edge of it, write down all the sentences that come up. Write a letter to it.

Art for soothing oneself:

Use art to return to your center and calm yourself. Make drawings just for fun. Leave your worries behind you, open your notebook on a blank page, and use colors and shapes that soothe you and do you good. Listen to pleasant music if you feel like it (2002, p. 174–176). (Free translation).

## Safe haven techniques

For treating trauma, security considerations are always paramount in order to avoid re-traumatizing the client. Many therapists use the visualization of a safe haven to turn to, in order to avoid dissociation in the course of treatment.[10] In art therapy, we can easily ask a patient to draw such a safe haven or even to make a three-dimensional model thereof. I am convinced that the conferring of an objective external reality to the safe haven reinforces its potential to secure and calm the patient. Jobin (2002) proposes her own version of it:

Healing space:

Draw a healing or recharging space. If you like, include the wounded child or your injury (…) Please create this space to your liking; it can be as much the core of a flower as a cave or the arms of an angel, or just soothing colours (2002, p. 188). (Free translation).

## Identity reconstruction techniques

There are a number of possible techniques for identity reconstruction purposes, as every client and interview are unique and art therapists tailor their interventions to the specific needs of their clients. The *life line drawing* exercise inspired by the life story method is a good choice. We ask clients to draw a long unfinished line on a large paper and to draw significant events of their life. This exercise can help to put the traumatic events in perspective by considering them in the broader perspective of a person's entire life. It can also be used to acknowledge positive events, achievements, confirming experiences, and moments when they could give and receive.[11]

## Personal integrity restoration techniques

Here as well, it is difficult to list all the possibilities, because there are a number of sound methods. Nonetheless, I would like to mention two original techniques that are particularly suited to restoring personal integrity. The first is the drawing or collage of a *positive future* to instill a sense of hope[12] and possibly alleviate the feeling of facing a bleak future, which is one of the frequent symptoms people encounter in PTSD.

The second one is Joyce Mills' (2006) wonderful experience with the 'bowl of light'. First developed and used with Hawaian communities in the aftermath of a hurricane, it was subsequently used with children in a number of schools in Hawaii. When her grant expired, more than 4,000 'bowls of light' had been created in the Westside community in Hawaii. After telling a Hawaiian legend, the activity continued with the creation of a three-dimensional 'bowl of light', which, according to the author, increases the healing potential on conscious and unconscious levels. It can also help to rebuild and increase self-esteem and self-appreciation. The 'bowl of light' can also be drawn, and/or a therapeutic ritual can be performed to complete the experience. This method is detailed in Appendix B.[13]

## Notes

1  See Asmundson, G. J. G. *et al.* (2002). *Op. Cit.* and Otis, J. D. *et al.* (2003). *Op. Cit.*
2  Jacobson, M., 1994: *Op. Cit.*
3  Jacobson, M. (1994). *Op. Cit.*, p. 48.
4  See chapter 4.
5  See Levine, P. 2015, 2009, 2005, 1997.
6  See Carey, L. (2006). *Op. Cit.;* McCarthy, D. (2006): *Op. Cit.* and Lacroix, L. (2002): *Op. Cit.*
7  See Frey, D. (2006). Puppetry interventions for traumatized clients. In: Carey, L. *Expressive and Creative Arts Methods for Trauma Survivors*. London and Philadelphia, PA: Jessica Kingsley.
8  Carey, L. (2006). *Op. Cit.*
9  See also Hamel, J. (1997). 'L'approche gestaltiste en thérapie par l'art'. *Revue Québécoise de Gestalt, 2(1)*, 130–147.
10  See Jacobson, M., 1994; Rothschild, B., 2000; Scaer, R., 2001 and Carey, L., 2006.
11  Carey, L. (2006). *Op. Cit.*
12  Carey, L. (2006). *Op. Cit.*, p. 36.
13  Mills, J. (2006) The bowl of light: A story-craft for healing. In: Carey, L. (2006) *Expressive and Creative Arts Methods for Trauma Survivors*, 207–213. London and Philadelphia, PA: Jessica Kingsley.

# Part III
# Theoretical Concepts

# 6    Hypotheses About Art Therapy Effectiveness

*Johanne Hamel*

Based on my clinical experience, my readings on the treatment of PTSD, the work of art therapists and my clinical research, I have a few hypotheses about the reasons for the effectiveness of art therapy in the treatment of PTSD and chronic pain. I singled out six effectiveness factors in art therapy:

- The power of images to facilitate abreaction
- Right brain stimulation
- Isomorphism
- Objectification
- Containment
- Security

## The power of images to facilitate abreaction

Often, images created in art therapy sessions will produce abreaction, an expression of repressed emotions. The visual stimulation at the same time as the motor stimulation produced by the movements on paper seem conductive to emotional expression. Repressed emotions are dissociated from the conscious experience of clients. Reclaiming what is unconscious is the way to wholeness.

Art therapy also makes it possible to use even just a part of an image (for example, a colour present in the environment during a trauma) to access repressed or forgotten elements. Almost any art therapy approach, in a safe therapeutic context, can bring back trauma or abuse or repressed emotions if they are present in the experience of the client.

We can understand even better the power of images if we consider Levine's theory. As you will see in chapter 7, images are part of any experience according to Levine's SIBAM model. SIBAM as an acronym means sensation, image, behavior, affect, and meaning. Attention to one of the elements of the model gives access to the others, so images can be used to find missing, dissociated or unconscious elements.

Furthermore, if there is no conscious image, drawing any interoceptive physical sensation (sensation), an intense emotion (affect) or even a repeated involuntary movement (behavior) are all strategies that, according to clinical observations, allow for the reintegration of all the elements of the experience (SIBAM model), give access to meaning making and/or to procedural trauma memory (see chapter 7). Intense emotions not available yet become accessible. Through this self-expression, relaxation can be sustained.

## Right brain stimulation

Images are the language of the psyche, and especially of the implicit processes of the right brain. *Left brain* and *right brain* are actually oversimplification of the hemispheric specialization. Today in neurosciences, we rather talk about *explicit* and *implicit* neuronal pathways. However, it is true that the left side of the brain contains more specialized neuronal pathways connected to the use of language, of rational thought, and planification (explicit information), while the right brain is more specialized in images, emotional reactions, and intuition (implicit information); the right brain apprehends reality as a whole.

A person *freezes* when trapped in a traumatic situation from which it is impossible to escape.[1]Van der Kolk (1996) has demonstrated that it is the left side of the brain, responsible for speech and language, and especially the Broca's area, which freezes, while the right side of the brain shows more activity, especially in the limbic area and the amygdala. Now, we know that art turns on the right side of the brain. Images are conjured in the right brain, and in PTSD, they are associated with deep emotions. These emotions inhibit the functioning of the cerebral cortex (left brain). Traumatic memories stored as images in the right brain become accessible through drawing and painting.

When trauma images become a tangible reality on paper, the words to talk about the trauma are found once again. A reconnection between the right brain and the left brain then occurs. PTSD symptoms such as nightmares, re-experiencing of the events, emotional distress, and hypervigilance decrease or disappear following their creation on paper. Golub (1985) mentions the case of a veteran whose recurring nightmares ceased after having painted them. Morgan and Johnson (1995) also reported the case of two veterans whose nightmares were reduced in intensity and frequency after drawing them (see the study below).

## Isomorphism

Janie Rhyne describes isomorphism as follows:

> 'The way we perceive visually is directly related to how we think and feel; the correlation becomes apparent when we represent our perceptions with art materials. The central figures we depict emerge from a diffuse background and give us clues as to what is central to our lives. The way we use lines, shapes and colours in relation to

each other, and the space we put them in indicates something about how we pattern our lives'.

(1984, 8–9)

This means that whatever we create on the paper is a projection of us, a reflection of a part of our experience. If we add to the isomorphism principle the fact that artistic expression often precedes verbal expression, as art often reveals aspects of the patient's experience that he did not consciously grasp or wanted to represent voluntarily, it is understood that art offers unique opportunities for intense but repressed experiences to reveal themselves.

According to Johnson (1987), problems in accessing traumatic events when there is denial or amnesia are largely attributable to the neural encoding process of the event. He points out that traumatic memories in flashbacks or nightmares, for instance, are exact replica of the event down to the smallest detail as if they were photographs.[2] Unlike normal memories, which vary a little each time they are recalled, traumatic events are always recalled exactly as they initially were. A memory encoded this way is inflexible: it is completely separated from the next one and can be accessed only by similar situations recalling the unconscious or forgotten event. Normal memory reconstitutes the elements using a hierarchical system of similar stimuli. It is more flexible and is based on associative links between phenomena.

For Johnson, everything happens as if – in moments of terror – the otherwise developed cognitive function is overwhelmed, and the event is recorded in a photographic form, as a global memory not conceptually integrated with other memories through the normal associative links. This memory cannot therefore be digested, worked on, or transformed like any other aspects of memory. As mentioned earlier, recent discoveries in neuro-imaging confirm the deactivation of the temporal lobe responsible for language and thought, specifically the Broca's area, and the activation of the limbic system in which traumatic images are encoded.[3] These memories have a highly visual component but also highly sensorimotor qualities. Using verbal and discursive forms of thought interferes with access to these unconscious thoughts, which would explain why hypnosis, dreamwork, and free associations are used in psychoanalysis.[4]

Many authors consider that a visual medium such as art facilitates access to traumatic images and memories.[5] Howard also refers to *isomorphism* to describe this visual connection between art and traumatic memory: both are a visual sensory process. She sees images as mental contents with sensory qualities that are distinct from mental activity, which is purely verbal or abstract.[6]

## Objectification

Moreover, these authors[7] consider that using art materials to externalize traumatic images helps to distance a client from the painful content intensity of the internalized image, thereby enabling him to have a sense of control and to preserve his integrity. 'Because art is concrete and external, the patient can discuss the image of a feeling rather than emotion itself' (Howard, 1990, 81).

Lambert and Simard, speaking of a population of sexually abused women, refer to 'a power allowing to distancing oneself from too strong emotions':

'Art therapy offers women tools to safely express strong emotions of anger or sadness (having a destructive potential). It allows catharsis without acting out, in a safe manner. As invasive emotions are drawn on paper, art therapy also allows, if necessary, to distance oneself from them' (Free translation).

(Lambert and Simard, 1997, 218)

## Containment

Artistic production as part of a safe therapeutic relationship also has a containment function, or *temenos*. [8] I personally consider that the projection of an image onto a physical and tangible medium (paper), of a specific size and external to oneself, makes one feel like leaving behind a part of one's experience on paper and to perceive it as contained within clear – therefore secure – boundaries (paper). This, in itself, has a soothing effect. In some way, the image becomes *contained within the paper* and no longer *contained within the memory*.

Morgan and Johnson (1995) observed a similar effect in the treatment of nightmares in soldiers suffering from PTSD:

'The "canvas" provides a transitional space in which memory and current reality can mix within the perceived control of the subject, so that the ability to integrate previous self-images with the traumatic event is enhanced'.

(Morgan and Johnson, 1995, p. 244)

## Security

That experience with two soldiers[9] would tend to confirm the hypothesis that drawing nightmares does not retraumatize the client, while the use of written language might do so. Morgan and Johnson (1995) worked with two veterans with nightmares, comparing the effect of drawing with that of writing. In a 12-weeks intervention in which drawing and writing alternated three weeks on and three weeks off, both subjects reported a decrease in the frequency and intensity of nightmares during the weeks that they drew them upon waking up, while their nightmares worsened in the weeks when they noted them down as soon as they woke up. The statistical study using an Anova test to measure the differences between the two conditions showed significant differences in the frequency of recurring nightmares, in their intensity, and in the startle response upon waking up, as well as in the difficulty with getting back to sleep. There was no significant difference between the two subjects. They would explain this research result by the isomorphism between art and nightmares. It is very likely that one could achieve the same outcomes with drawings of flashbacks or traumatic memories.

In addition, in art therapy, the patient controls his or her experience in many ways in the context of a safe, helping relationship. First, the choice of the medium allows for control, as it will allow a greater or lesser emotional distance in a very effective way. As mentioned earlier, the art media have a psychological impact that the art therapist knows and can use together with the patient.

Furthermore, it is the patient who draws or paints, thus acting out the experience; she or he can control the pace, content, and depth of his experience.[10] Through the patient's control over her or his experience, the intrusive re-experiencing is transformed into mere memories.[11]

I do not think that these hypotheses are comprehensive in explaining the effectiveness of art therapy for treating PTSD and chronic pain; research could help us to learn more. The case studies presented in the next chapters will illustrate this *lively effectiveness,* as Carl Jung[12] stated about art.

## Notes

1 Levine, P. (1997). *Op. Cit.*

2 About this, the author cites Van der Kolk, B. *et al.* (1984).

3 Van der Kolk, B. A. (1996). The body keeps the score: approaches to the psychobiology of posttraumatic stress disorder. In: Van der Kolk, B. A., McFarlane, A. C. & Weisaeth, L. (1996). *Traumatic Stress: the Effects of Overwhelming Experience on Mind, Body, and Society,* pp. 214–241. New York, NY: Guilford Press.

4 According to Johnson, D. R. (1987). 'Perspective: The role of the creative arts therapies in the diagnosis and treatment of psychological trauma'. *The Arts in Psychotherapy, An International Journal, 14(1),* 7–14.

5 See among others: Johnson, D. R. (1987); Howard, R. (1990), and Lambert, J. & Simard, P. (1997).

6 Howard, R. (1990). 'Art therapy as an isomorphic intervention in the treatment of a client with post-traumatic stress disorder'. *The American Journal of Art Therapy, 28(3),* 79–87.

7 See: Johnson, D. R. (1987); Howard, R. (1990) and Lambert, J. & Simard, P. (1997).

8 Duchastel, A. (2005). *Op. Cit.*

9 See: Morgan, C. A. & Johnson, D. R. (1995). *Op. Cit.*

10 See Howard, R. (1990) as well as Lambert, J. & Simard, P. (1997).

11 Johnson, D. R. (1987). 'Perspective: The role of the creative arts therapies in the diagnosis and treatment of psychological trauma'. *The Arts in Psychotherapy, An International Journal, 14(1),* 7–14.

12 Jung, C. (1993). *La Guérison Psychologique.* Geneva: Georg, 6th ed.

# 7 Dissociative Processes in Post-Traumatic Stress Disorders

*Johanne Hamel*

According to the DSM-V (2013), the presence of dissociative symptoms is part of the diagnostic criteria of post-traumatic stress disorder (PTSD) and of acute stress disorders. Indeed, for the authors who will be discussed here, dissociation is at the heart of PTSD and explains its chronicity. Scaer (2001) has consistently seen dissociation in PTSD. This chapter will address Levine's (1997) theoretical perspectives on *somatic dissociation* and the SIBAM model, those of van der Kolk (1996) on *somatic memory* and the limits of talk therapy, as well as those of Scaer on *procedural memory*. These concepts are important to highlight how somatic art therapy can be effective in treating PTSD and chronic pain.

## Levine's somatic dissociation: The SIBAM model

Levine explains somatic dissociation as trauma being trapped inside the body. PTSD, he argues, is fundamentally a biological response to trauma, a response that is highly activated, incomplete and frozen in time.

Levine thinks that when you are unable to defend yourself when a trauma occurs or to prevent an accident, unfinished defensive actions become blocked and stored in the nervous system as non-discharged energy. For him, trauma is essentially an interrupted action that the body needs to complete.[2]

The SIBAM model:

He developed a very useful model: the SIBAM dissociation model. SIBAM is the acronym for sensation, image, behavior, affect, and meaning. Levine[3] postulates that these elements are dissociated during traumatic experiences, which results in different forms of dissociation, while other elements are associated, which leads to different forms of re-experiencing (like flashbacks for instance). Here are two examples from Babette Rothschild (2000):

- Association between affect and sensation and dissociation from image, behavior and meaning:

Clients with anxiety and panic attacks might talk persistently about disturbing physical sensations and resulting fear (affect). It might be difficult or impossible for them to identify what they heard or saw that triggered the anxiety (image), what they need to do to reduce the anxiety (behavior), or what the fear actually stems from (meaning).

• Association between image and affect and dissociation from sensation, behavior, and meaning:

Clients trapped in visual flashbacks will shuttle between the images and terror (affect), blocked in their ability to feel their body in the present (sensation), move in a way that would break the spell (behavior), or put the memory into context (meaning) (2000, p. 69–70).

The SIBAM model allows the associated elements and the dissociated ones to be identified then helps the missing elements to be gradually reintegrated into consciousness. Images being one of these elements, they can be used in somatic art therapy to help to find the missing elements. Given my clinical experience, as well as Levine's (1997), Scaer's (2001), and Rothschild's (2000), findings indicate that *attention to one of the elements of the model gives access to others.* Once reintegration occurs, many symptoms will disappear.

## Van der Kolk's somatic memory

Bessel van der Kolk (1994) describes how trauma disrupts the hormonal stress management system, as well as the entire nervous system, preventing the integration of traumatic memories into consciousness. He explains the complex physiological processes by which trauma memories remain in the non-verbal, subconscious, subcortical regions of the brain (amygdala, thalamus, hippocampus, and hypothalamus, identified as the right brain by art therapists), where they are not accessible to the frontal lobes, i.e. to areas of the brain associated with understanding, thinking, and reasoning (identified as the left brain by art therapists). Van der Kolk (cited in Carey, 2006) explains how neuroimaging scans have shown that when people remember traumatic events, the left frontal cortex stops functioning, especially the Broca's area, which is responsible for speech and language. In contrast, right hemisphere areas associated with emotional states and autonomic arousal, including the amygdala, are activated. Therefore, when people remember traumatic events, the frontal lobe becomes dysfunctional, and they experience thinking and speaking limitations as a result.[4]

For van der Kolk, it is the body that controls our response to trauma, not our mind; consequently, trauma treatment requires that therapists consider the body as well. Once you can do what you could not do during the trauma, once you can take the necessary action to protect yourself, and once you are able to return to your center and refocus on a solid organismic basis, you will change (1994, p. 263–265).

Van der Kolk clearly believes that words alone cannot integrate the disorganized sensations and actions that have become stuck in trauma, but also that talking through the trauma experience is important. Talk is relevant and, in fact, essential for traumatized patients who do not really know what happened to them, who were too young to understand what happened, whom no one listened to or believed, or who need help to make sense of what happened. Even though he describes his own therapy as still very verbal, he maintains that words alone are not enough.[5]

The importance given to the body comes from his belief in a somatic memory, a concept familiar to body therapists that validates their own experiences with traumatized patients (Rothschild, 2000; Sykes Wylie, 2004; Carey, 2006).

One example reported by Lindy, Green & Grace (cited in Rothschild, 2000) demonstrates the somatic re-enactment of a traumatic event. One woman's recurring somatic and behavioral re-flashback involved a persistent, debilitating symptom of urinary urgency causing repeated, unnecessary trips to the restroom. Both symptom and behavior developed following a restaurant fire where her life was literally spared by an empty bladder; indeed, her friends had died trapped in the restroom. It seemed as though she was reliving the moment when her decision not to go to the bathroom proved to be crucial.

This example poignantly illustrates how someone can act in ways that seem to make no sense unless you know the trauma history. However, the nature of somatic re-enactment becomes clear when the missing pieces of information are supplied. It is possible that certain unexplained physical symptoms that puzzle doctors and plague patients could be incidents of somatic re-enactment (Rothschild, 2000, p. 71).

For van der Kolk, therapists need to help patients to feel their self-efficacy as a functioning biological organism and to restore a sense of inner security. Therapists pay attention to feelings, sensations, and inner physical impulses for the patient to be able to familiarize himself with her or his feelings and rely on her or his inner experience, as well as restore her or his relationship with the physical self.[6]

For Lois Carey, art therapist, it is clear that a holistic approach is required, one that is based on mind-body integration, where creative arts therapies have a legitimate place in the treatment of mental health disorders and play a vital role in treating trauma. She wrote the following:

> Although van der Kolk's recommendations remain controversial in the scientific community, he validates what many seasoned clinicians have recognized for a long time: that creative arts therapies, whether sandplay therapy, art, drama, music, somatic or dance therapies, massage, yoga, and the martial arts offer considerable benefits to clients who have not fully benefited from traditional verbal therapies.
>
> (2006, p. 25)

## Scaer's procedural memory

As mentioned previously, Scaer believes that myofascial pain comes either from the procedural memory of regional muscle tension patterns at the time of an impact (in an accident), or from a trauma having threatened the life of the individual.[7] He says:

> In our chronic pain program, we invariably see that the patients' unconscious posture reflects not only their pain, but also the experience of the traumatic event that produced the pain. The asymmetrical postural patterns, held in procedural memory, almost always reflect the body's attempt to move away from the injury or threat that caused the injury.
>
> (Sacer, 2001, 106)

Scaer worked with many motor vehicle accident (MVA) victims and studied the unexplainable pains and the many symptoms of whiplash. He sees the whiplash syndrome as not arising from any structural injuries to the spine, jaw, or brain, but rather as the result of trauma.[8]

For Scaer, PTSD symptoms are explained by a repetitive neurological feedback loop called the kindling process, which is predisposed by the freeze response. This response leads to a state of sustained neurovegetative overactivation and to alternation of the autonomic nervous system between the overactivation and a state of dissociation. The process unfolds as follows: triggers from either the internal state or external cues regularly activate the amygdala, which in turn would interpret the resulting emotions and the memories thus activated as threatening and would again generate overactivation. As a result, all the common re-experiencing and overactivation phenomena are observed.[9]

By repeating over and over again, the neurobiological loops create a self-perpetuating pathway, and the overactivation incidents reoccur more and more readily, i.e. the triggers become more and more pervasive.

Triggers are obviously associated with trauma, i.e. the trauma memory. These memories are also linked to the sensory organs involved in the traumatic experience, which generates repetitive loops of the somatic symptoms representative of the intense sensory experience at the time of the trauma. For example, the specific distribution of the muscles involved in the myofascial pain will be the one of the contracted muscles in response to the velocity changes in the accident; these continue to contract when overactivation occurs or a trauma-related memory arises.[10]

This process provides a unitary hypothesis for the myriad symptoms of whiplash. It also provides a model for the concept of somatization, one of the more prominent comorbid conditions seen in PTSD (Scaer, 2001, p. 54).

Scaer reports a remarkable example of somatic dissociation seen in a MVA victim treated for chronic pain. Almost the entire skin of this young lady's forearm had been torn off in the accident. The sensation in the grafted skin never returned to normal, but she developed increasingly vague, hard-to-describe intense aching pain that was resistant to all treatments. The pain was associated with myofascial pain in the shoulder. Scaer noticed that the young woman was totally unaware of her unconscious posture of total rejection and dissociation of her entire left arm, even when looking in a mirror. When shown a photograph of herself, however, she became aware of it; with trauma therapy and postural education, the pain gradually disappeared as her posture approached a more normal status.[11]

It is a good example of an unconscious posture reflecting not only the pain, but also the experience of the traumatic event that produced the pain. The asymmetrical postural patterns, held in procedural memory, reflected the body's attempt to move away from the injury or threat that caused the injury.

By the pictorial representation of the physical sensation in the aching part of the body, somatic art therapy makes it possible to directly access the procedural memory and the intense feeling of threat, which could then be released. This releasing allows the easing of the tension associated with the procedural memory: the body can finally relax. An example will be given in chapter 12.

## Notes

1  SIBAM stands for sensation, image, behavior, affect, and meaning.
2  Sykes Wylie, M. (2004). *Op. Cit.*
3  Cited in Rothschild, B. (2000). *The Body Remembers. The Psychophysiology of Trauma and Trauma Treatment.* New York, NY: USA: W. W. Norton & Co.
4  Carey, L. (2006). *Op. Cit.*
5  Carey, L. (2006). *Op. Cit.*, 24–25.
6  Van der Kolk, B. 1994, cited in Sykes Wylie, M. (2004). *Op. Cit.*
7  Scaer, R. C. (2001). *The Body Bears the Burden. Trauma, Dissociation, and Disease.* Binghamton, NY: The Haworth Medical Press.
8  Scaer, R. (2001). *Op. Cit.*
9  Scaer, R. (2001). *Op. Cit.*
10  Scaer, R. (2001). *Op. Cit.*
11  Scaer, R. (2001). *Op. Cit.*

# 8 Neuroscience and Somatic Art Therapy

## Emotional Memory Reconsolidation

*Sophie Boudrias*

'People have a huge need to feel their pain. Very often pain is the beginning of a great deal of awareness'.

Arnold Mindell

Emotional memory reconsolidation is a process that can be conducted through various psychotherapeutic approaches. Coherence therapy, Gestalt therapy, emotion-focused therapy sand play therapy, as well as creative therapy approaches particular facilitate the activation and transformation of emotional memories (Ecker, Ticic, and Hulley, 2012). This chapter aims to provide an insight into and illustrate the specific contribution of art therapy, and particularly of somatic art therapy, to facilitate the emotional memory reconsolidation process.

## Emotional memory

An emotional memory (or emotional learning) is an implicit memory that can be reactivated with or without the input of the declarative/explicit memory, the latter allowing to recall the initiating events of an emotional memory. Therefore, emotional memories impact affects and human behaviours often even without any consciousness of the connection between the two. As an example, one can feel fear when one's nose detects a specific odour, but without consciously attaching it to the fragrance one's assailant was wearing during a past trauma. Just as the procedural-implicit memory guides our body without us having to consciously direct it (for example, riding a bicycle, the learning being well consolidated) our emotional memories determine our spontaneous responses and our behaviours, very often despite our conscious will.

The veto right of emotional memories over our conscious will likely has a survival function, which may explain the persistence of these memories. Actually, in a situation of imminent threat, there would be little point in engaging into lengthy considerations about different potential actions. Our response is therefore quick and spontaneous in situations where we experience fear, our body taking immediate action to protect itself, by a fight-or-flight response.

Emotions and emotional memories have a physical component etched into the body. Somatic art therapy uses this component to access emotional memories from the body image, sensations and physical symptoms, as represented visually by the individual.

## Memory consolidation and reconsolidation

Consolidating a memory (or learning) means to move it from an actively working memory (or short-term memory) to the state of long-term memory that Lewis (1979) also calls 'inactive memory'. Consolidation and memory recall capability are facilitated by various factors, including the associated emotional weight and the memorization background (location, lighting, noises, odors, etc.). It has long been known that images and drawings promote the memorization processes (Shepard, 1967; Wammes, Meade, and Fernandes 2016). However, Ottarsdottir (2018) observed that drawings contribute not only to memorization and learning but also to the processing of emotions.

It might be tempting to believe that memory operates as a camera recording scenes in their entirety and replaying them identically during memory recall. In fact, it is not the case. Our memories are first constructed, then reconstructed (or reconsolidated) whenever we are revisiting them. A consolidated memory (long-term or inactive memory) that is recalled or reactivated in the short-term memory will be reconsolidated subsequently, often partly altered and not in its entirety.

The reconsolidation process therefore reactivates the target memory so that it can return to a labile state, allowing it to be altered (Nader, Schafe, and Le Doux, 2000). This flexibility allows the updating of the memory by activating a counter-experience simultaneously, in other words by recording a new learning that contradicts the old memory. To be able to transform an emotional memory associated with a phobia or a trauma, the old emotional memory first needs to be rekindled, and so does the affect that it is composed of. This process of updating then transforms how an individual feels or reacts about the same memory recall cues that previously activated the emotional memory, whether consciously or not.

The reconsolidation therapy (Brunet, Orr, Tremblay, Robertson, Nader, and Pitman, 2008), conducted in particular for treating post-traumatic stress disorder, uses a beta-blocking agent called propranolol, for the purpose of blocking the reconsolidation process of the trauma memory. One might therefore assume that you need only to take the medication to heal, therefore saving yourself from reopening old wounds. Still, the drug effectiveness is actually conditional on rekindling first the emotional memory and thus the associated affect.

## Emotional avoidance

The reconsolidation of an emotional memory is conditional upon activating the experiential and emotional dimensions thereof (Ecker et al., 2012).

However, recounting memories, without reliving them, will instead activate the declarative episodic memory. Therefore, emotional avoidance keeps emotional memories intact, the latter somehow replaying on a loop, with no chance of being updated by the newly acquired learnings. To illustrate this phenomenon, we can visualize a black box in which emotional memories are embedded, cut out from new experiences that are completely contrary to them. Refusing to open this black box would be refusing to transform it.

Cognitive learning (declarative semantic memory) alone has not been able to alter emotional learning; the two contradictory learnings (or memories) then continue to operate in parallel, being activated in turn from an inner competition mechanism (Ecker, 2012). The coexistence of the two memories might also generate a sense of inner conflict or being torn apart, which might be responsible for the request for counselling. As an example, if a woman seeks to stop going into jealous rages, specifying that she 'cannot help it', there is little point in suggesting to her that such a behaviour could jeopardize her relationship.

On a cognitive level, she is aware of that. However, such a behaviour being maintained by emotional memories, it is essential to address the affect and not only the mind, in order to be able to transform these memories. Now, images and colours have the property to arouse the affect, often more than words alone, as the right brain plays a major role in terms of both the processing of uncomfortable emotions and thinking by means of images and metaphors (Schore, 2008).

## The prerequisites in psychotherapy

In experiments conducted on animals with regard to memory reconsolidation, the memory to be reconsolidated will first be generated in a laboratory. For example, fear is induced in a rat, and this will then become the target memory to be reconsolidated. However, in psychotherapy, the target memory is not pre-defined. Thus, the *symptom* about which the client is complaining and wants to see eliminated must be identified beforehand with his help. Next, it is important to be very clear about the underlying *schema* of such a symptom, in other words the 'pro-symptom position' of the client (Ecker *et al.*, 2012). Finally, one must identify or create a *counter-experience* that will enable a new learning to be consolidated. The table below provides examples of the three components to be specified before conducting the reconsolidation process itself.

## Identifying the symptom

Hamel defines (See chapter 1) somatic art therapy as follows: 'Somatic art therapy provides access to soma through two-dimensional or three-dimensional representations (drawing, painting, clay, etc.) of the physical sensation felt subjectively', p. 8. Through such an approach, images first allow to identify the

*Table 8.1* Three components to be specified before conducting the reconsolidation process.

| Symptom | Schema | Counter-Experience |
|---|---|---|
| Self-assertiveness problem (psychological symptom) | 'If I offer an opinion that is different than that of others, I will experience rejection and sadness'. | I hear a friend offering an opinion that is very different from other people and I am surprised that the others feel grateful for his sharing, and still appreciate him. |
| Recurring headaches (physical symptom) | 'Physical pain is the only decent reason to refuse to fulfill a responsibility (like my *marital duties*) without feeling guilty'. | I refuse to have sex with my husband, although I am feeling fine, and I feel accepted despite my refusal. So I feel more free, and I no longer see sexuality as a *duty*, but as a choice. |

symptom and the schema by which it is maintained, for example, by becoming aware of a visual gestalt within the created images, or through what is revealed by the creative process itself. In Hamel's four-quadrants method (See chapter 10), the first drawing refers to identifying the symptom (quadrant #1), by representing the physical symptom itself on a piece of paper sheet or in a quadrant within a giant mandala.

In art therapy, as with any other psychotherapy approach, the client starts by describing his symptoms to the therapist. Somatic art therapy has the advantage of enabling access to soma and to the way in which the client represents the symptom. As a matter of fact, the physical or somatic symptoms are invisible when they are felt in the body. The client thus creates his own representation of the reality he feels, that being an image of his inner world. Somatic art therapy therefore makes it possible to access this representation and to make it externally visible through plastic arts. This causes the client to make the effort to accurately feel the symptom, making sure his representation is consistent with his feeling. For instance, the client will have to identify where the pain is felt in his body, to pick up a colour to represent it, to identify its size or intensity, etc. This representation gives access to additional information, which the client would neither necessarily verbalize spontaneously nor feel nor become aware of in talk therapy mode. From the moment that the representation takes shape, engaging in an intervention is made possible, for instance to further explore the underlying schema.

### Identifying a symptom: case example

In the following example, the client arrived at a counselling session to address a sensation she had recently experienced at work. The circumstances associated with the symptom onset were first explored verbally with her. She was not going through anything stressful at the time. So I suggested a focusing exercise to better feel the sensation and visualize it. During the exercise, she described the sensation as follows: 'It feels like my chest and my head are constantly vibrating and I hear a humming sound. I feel shrouded and squeezed... it is hard to say'. Thus, I invited her to picture that sensation in her mind (See Figure 8.1).

This client's symptom was located at the 'contact boundary', in other words at the metaphorical place of exchanges between the organism and the environment (Masquelier-Savatier, 2017, 63). Imagining the sensation led her to get in touch with an aspect not identified while verbally describing her sensation, that she now identified as *the world outside weighing on me*. So, I suggested to picture that *outside world weighing on her*, which she did using the red colour.

## Identifying the schema

In order to identify the schema underlying the symptom, two highly successful techniques are the amplification of symptoms and symptom deprivation (Ecker *et al.*, 2012). Using these two techniques alternatively

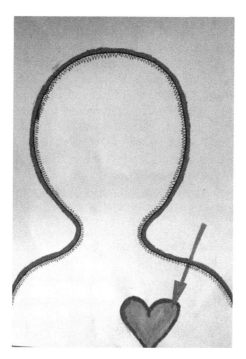

*Figure 8.1* The symptom, 12 inches x 18 inches (30.5 cm x 45 cm). Oil pastels, soft pastel, and coloured pencils. Pressure and vibration at the contact boundary. The arrow and the heart shape were added during the process.

also makes it possible to have a clear sense of both the effects of the symptom (including those that the individual might unconsciously seek), as well as those of the lack of symptoms (including those that the individual may unconsciously dread). Art therapy makes it possible to amplify the symptom, for example, by reproducing repetitively a line or a shape, or to amplify one element to better get in touch with it, until the underlying schema emerges. The symptom might also be actually withdrawn from the image, for example, by partly cutting out an image, in order to perceive the impacts of its absence, both visually and emotionally. Then it might be added back to ensure comparing the effects and the felt sense of both experiences.

As somatic art therapy requires getting involved in a creative process, the body is engaged into action. This engagement makes it possible for unconscious emotional memories to arise. Unconscious movements, visual lapsus, or body language slips, as well as any affects arising from the process then bring the symptom's function to light. The schema then becomes explicit and is made accessible to consciousness. At that point, the individual no longer perceives herself or himself as a powerless victim of her or his symptom and instead becomes aware that her or his symptom conveys a part of herself or himself or her or his own needs or fears. Although this kind of increasing awareness might be painful for the ego, it might also re-instill hopes of recovery, as the individual then becomes aware of his own power over the symptom.

In art therapy, images and body engagement bypass the conscious mind and the defense mechanisms that maintain emotional avoidance. Indeed, images are an indirect way of communicating that is protective for the ego, as one does not always refer directly to oneself in art therapy, but often rather refers to characters, animals, shapes, colours, and other elements that make up the images.

In the four-quadrants method (see chapter 10), the second drawing (quadrant #2) could also allow to specify the necessity schema and the origins of the symptom, as the client is asked to represent the very first recollection of the onset of the symptom.

## Symptom amplification: case example

The amplification of a symptom through somatic art therapy is shown in the following example. Figure 8.2 is based on the drawing from Figure 8.1, used during the same session with the client. In order for the client to further explore her or his symptom and understand its function, I suggested the selection of a small section of the first drawing to be enlarged on a different sheet of paper, as though it was viewed under a microscope. This is a Gestalt art therapy technique for amplification or exaggeration (Hamel, 1997). The client spontaneously selected an area located between the neck and the shoulder, then she reproduced it, visually enhancing what

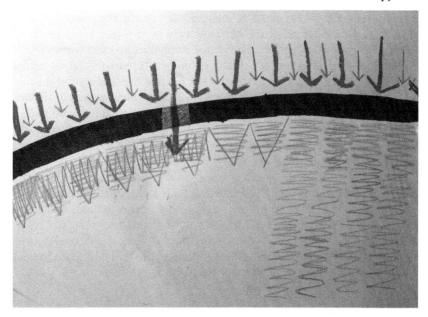

*Figure 8.2* Amplification of the symptom, 8½ inches x 11 inches (21.6 cm x 28 cm). Oil pastels, coloured pencils, and gouache. The arrow that is cutting through and the void within the black line were added during the process.

was shown in red, using arrows. While tracing zigzag lines within the body shape, she felt that the zigzagging movement went from left to right, pointing down to the inner area. By amplifying the red arrows exerting pressure, using repetition, she felt that they were seeking entry, whereas amplifying the black line (as a result of going over it again and self-identifying with the line by *giving it a voice*), she felt that the black line was denying entry, which resulted in a sense of vibration towards the inner area.

The black line reminded her of a hard and thick whale skin. The metaphors expressed or represented by clients often are rich gateways to access their subjective experience (Modell, 2003). Therefore, I further explored the client's metaphor, verbally this time, asking her how important it was for the whale to have thick skin. She stated that it prevented the arrows from piercing through and causing wounds, and that led to further explore the image regarding what would happen if ever it were pierced by an arrow.

The client first created a space within the dark line area, then she drew a red arrow pointing to the inner area. By transposing this arrow onto her body shape (Figure 8.1), the client became aware that it would pierce straight to her heart, and this led her to feel and express a sense of sadness, specifically with respect to her partner's behavior towards her. She made a connection between the process conducted during the session and the fact that she generally works hard at maintaining control both over her own emotions and actions and over her environment, in order to avoid being moved by what she experiences, in fear of being hurt and feel sorrow.

Therefore, her schema was phrased as follows: 'I must not let myself be touched by what upsets me. I must keep control because letting go and letting myself be touched means I will feel hurt, and I certainly do not want to feel sorrow'. To allow the arrow to get to her heart could seem counter-intuitive, given that it is hurtful. Yet that is exactly what was needed for her to be able to deal with the avoidance of symptoms: letting herself be touched and feel sorrow.

During the session, the client felt sorrow and expressed it in a safe context, which may have contributed to deconstruct the fear around that emotion. Her acceptance to feel provided information about her own needs and about the impact of her partner's behavior on her, which she had been seeking to control thus far in order to avoid getting hurt. So she experienced sorrow both from a safe place and as a process offering positive aspects, in terms of the information about herself, her needs and her love relationship.

## Symptom deprivation: case example

Figure 8.3 is from a client seeking counselling about a generalized anxiety disorder and recently diagnosed with other anxiety disorders (agoraphobia,

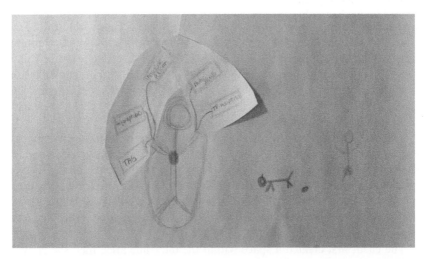

*Figure 8.3* The symptom: the tags, 18 inches x 24 inches (45 cm x 60 cm). Coloured pencils and oil pastels. The cutting out, the purple circle around the character, and the blue circle inside were added during the process.

social phobia, adjustment disorder, and performance anxiety) after consulting with a doctor. Upon arrival, she told me that she started thinking about all these psychological tags when going out to walk the dog for nature's needs, and that her daughter went out in the cold barely dressed in diapers. At that moment, she thought that all these tags would certainly prevent her to function normally. In order to better understand her symptom, I suggested that she represent this situation just as she had experienced it. Then she realized with surprise that the tags were not a part of her on the image, she was just holding them in her hand. When I questioned her about how she reacted to that observation, she said that it was like not wanting to let them go. This led to exploring the symptom's function, in other words the schema that caused her to stick to the tags.

Although anxiety can be experienced in the body, it is not so much the physical sensation itself that was worked on as a symptom during the session, but instead the client's need to preserve a self-image carrying diagnoses, despite the inconvenience involved.

In Figure 8.4, the client was invited to withdraw all tags in order to explore what would be the outcome of her letting go, which she did using scissors. Knowing that to her, the anxiety and the tags were responsible for her inability to handle the situation, I asked her how she viewed that situation with her daughter and her dog, now that the tags were gone. She then became emotional, answering: 'It means I am not a good mother, since my daughter went out dressed in diapers and got cold. I should have been able to handle both my daughter and my dog'. The fact that the symptom deprivation was represented and the deprivation was

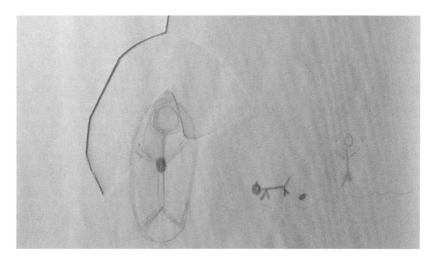

*Figure 8.4* Symptom deprivation: Letting go of the tags. 18 inches x 24 inches (45 cm x 60 cm). Colored pencils and oil pastels.

put into context visually with her daughter and her dog allowed her to access the schema necessitating the occurrence of the symptom: her anxiety (and her diagnoses) served the purpose of protecting her self-esteem in a context of high demands and self-judgments. As long as she held on to the tags, she could blame her perceived wrongdoings on them, as they were seen as external to her.

## Identifying or creating a counter-experience

A counter-experience is one that vividly contradicts the target emotional memory. It can be a past experience that is reactivated in the present, or a whole new experience to be created in the 'here and now'. The four-quadrants method shows the counter-experience (see chapter 10) in the third drawing (quadrant #4), in other words the drawing about the complete healing of the symptom.

In terms of memory reconsolidation, an imaginary experience is enough (Ecker *et al.*, 2012). The brain actually does not differentiate between an imaginary experience and an *actual* one, provided that the experience is properly visualized, put into context, and felt. In art therapy, creating images helps an individual to visualize and to put into context a counter-experience contained in other consolidated memories (long-term memory), or even to create a new one. Art therapy actually allows to create not only a cognitive knowledge rational in nature, but rather an actual counter-experience involving many feeling factors (visual, tactile, kinesthetic, emotional factors, etc.), in order to be able to compete with the target emotional memory, in an experiential dissonance.

## Counter-experience: case example

The client who created Figure 8.5 had been feeling extreme fatigue (symptom) for several months. Being a manager, she was receiving multiple requests both at work and in her personal life that she felt compelled to respond to. This symptom originated from an emotional memory that required from her to never take personal time for her self-care, otherwise she felt like a burden on others (schema). The roots of this memory dated back to her experience as a sick child, where coming from a large family, she felt guilty for her mother spending time with her at the hospital, while her brothers and sisters were deprived from maternal attendance.

The client started with drawing her symptom, stating that the depicted character *just feels the need to withdraw into its shell like a snail,* but *she* certainly did not want to do that. Once again using the client's sponta-neous metaphor as a gateway to access her subjective experience, I sug-gested that she create the snail using clay. First, the snail was portrayed with a large shell, and she described it as being very heavy. While

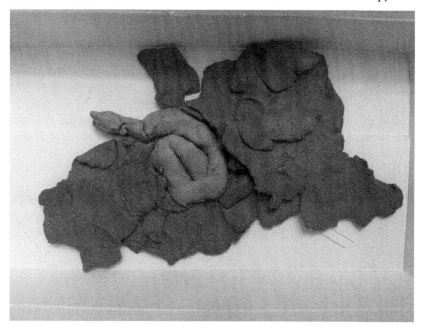

*Figure 8.5* Counter-experience: the snail recharging in nature (cross-sectional view), about 6 inches x 8 inches (15 cm x 20 cm). Clay.

holding the snail in her hand, stripping its shell off bit by bit, she got in touch with her vulnerability and started feeling compassion for it (therefore self-compassion for her own vulnerability). Then I asked her what it would need right now: *To seek refuge underground to feed and recharge.* Thus, she created such a nurturing and restful environment for the snail from the piece of clay previously used for the shell, then she breathed a long sigh of relief.

I invited the client to stay in tune with what the snail was now feeling. This allowed her to fully feel the counter-experience, in other words the well-being provided by such a recharging time, to ensure that it would override the guilt induced by the initial emotional memory. When she left, she stressed her determination to go home and lie down in her pajamas on the couch and wrap up in a warm blanket for the rest of the evening, admitting that it was long past due.

Thus, somatic art therapy allowed the client to work metaphorically starting from her fatigue symptom, literally and actually transforming an old way of protecting herself against a perceived threat by carrying a heavy shell, which led to a more appropriate attitude for her current context (nourishing earth), in other words accepting to rest and take care of herself with self-compassion.

## Facilitating the emotional memory reconsolidation process

With these three elements in place (symptom, schema, and counter-experience), the reconsolidation process starts by activating the emotional memory associated with the symptom, the memory thus returning to a labile state. Such flexibility lasts for a four-hour or five-hour time window (Nader et al., 2000; Ecker et al., 2012). It is during this timeframe that the counter-experience needs to be activated for the reconsolidation to occur. The juxtaposition of the two contradictory learnings creates an experiential dissonance that prompts the body to select which one of the two contradictory learnings needs to be maintained. Although we go through counter-experiences on a regular basis in everyday life, they often do not affect our emotional memories, as these might not necessarily be simultaneously activated. Actually, we even are often prone to keep them from rising, given the pain associated with them.

In art therapy, representing both the emotional memory and the counter-experience makes it possible to visually juxtapose both contradictory learnings (for example, on a single sheet divided into two sections or on two sheets placed side by side). That is why I usually do not recommend to my clients to use the back of their drawing, unless it has a specific purpose or a symbolic function for them. Hass-Cohen and Findlay (2009) have actually created a protocol that allows such visual juxtaposition for the purpose of memory reconsolidation.

In verbal psychotherapy, juxtaposition is repeated through alternating between emotional memory activation and counter-experience activation (Ecker *et al.*, 2012), given the linear nature of spoken language. In art psychotherapy, it is also possible to maintain (rather than repeat) an integrated representation (rather than a juxtaposition) of the two memories, because images have properties allowing to stay connected with many visual stimuli simultaneously. This is what the impact of the last drawing (quadrant #3) is about in the four-quadrants method (see chapter 10), as this step is about illustrating the transition between the symptom and healing, by borrowing visual elements from both drawings. The use of arts also makes it possible to transform the emotional memory image itself (symptom and/or schema) in the course of the process, into a representation of the counter-experience using the same plastic artwork, as illustrated in the last example.

In conclusion, somatic art therapy is a preferred approach for facilitating emotional memory reconsolidation. Engaging the body to creative action as well as the properties specific to images, metaphors, and the creative process are all powerful therapy tools, both for identifying and transforming emotional memories.

# 9 Somatic Heart Coherence and the Quantum Model

*Mylène Piché*

What do we really know about health and healing? While traditional medicine continues to astound us with unimaginable breakthroughs in terms of surgery and technological advances, I cannot help but notice that we are quite limited when it comes to therapeutic means. Despite giant leaps made by research over the past 50 years, it remains difficult for us to find the origins of many diseases that we want to eradicate. We need only to look at cancer, chronic diseases, multiple sclerosis, and orphan diseases to see the long road ahead before we find a cure for many pathologies. In the past, our medical model was focused on understanding the physical mechanisms involved in the onset of pain and disease. Today, we are witnessing the emergence of an 'integral medicine' (Goswami, 2013) that now focuses on the impact of the mind over the physical body.

This new healthcare model attempts to map the quantum mechanisms responsible for disease and healing. Deepak Chopra, one of the most renowned precursors in this field, is mainly responsible for educating the general public about what he defines as 'quantum healing' (Chopra, 2019, 2015, 2009). The basis of this approach lies in the pivotal role that consciousness plays over gene activation, and we are invited to look beyond the boundaries of our physical bodies to explain and treat the source of disease.

As this model is rooted in the field of quantum physics, it underlines the importance of paying attention to the energetic dimension which has precedence over *material* reality that we are aware of. Although invisible to the human eye, the design of this dimension is made of infinite waves of potentialities that are affected by our consciousness, our thoughts, and our emotions. We can picture this as an ocean of vibrational matter made of endless potentialities in an unmanifested form. This quantum ocean is actually where all the vibrational frequencies governing material manifestation lie, including health and disease.

For any potentiality to be experienced in the physical world, the corresponding wavelength needs to collapse (Goswami, 2013, 31). In other words, we must choose and extract a desired potentiality from the vibrational ocean in which it is immersed. But who makes such a *choice*? According to the quantum model, the observer who chooses to focus his consciousness on a given wavelength will trigger that collapsing. This will result in the manifestation of its contents to our physical reality. Now, it is important to understand that we cannot activate this collapsing mechanism from our *ordinary ego* as demonstrated by the quantum physicist Amit Goswami, author of *The Quantum Doctor* (2013).This crucial concept will be further explored in this chapter, as it supports the potential contribution that *somatic art therapy* can offer to the development of a new integrative medicine.

Based on this new paradigm, the physical world as we know it becomes a whole different matter. Just like Goswami, the epigeneticist Bruce Lipton, author of *The Biology of Belief (2016)*, demonstrates the significant roles played by consciousness, beliefs, and their corresponding vibrations in the manifestation of disease and health. His research, and those of other scientists, now invites us to review the relationship between this collapsing mechanism, our mind, and the *finished product* known as our body. Their view is closely related to the fundamental principles of *somatic art therapy* and corroborates many of the methods used by Johanne Hamel to deal with the origins of physical symptoms.

Now, do we really know what it means to act on 'vibrational matter' while it is still in the form of wavelengths and potentialities?

## Connection with our source design

Our organism is naturally endowed with healing properties. When we cut ourselves, it is fascinating to see the body's capacity to self-repair without relying on any external procedure. We all have experienced the power and the intelligence of this invisible *source consciousness* designed to repair cuts, heal infections, or resolve uncomfortable physical symptoms without paying it direct attention. However, we have collectively lost trust in the source design of our consciousness and in our body's inherent capacity to self-repair, believing somehow that healing is mostly a matter for machines and drugs.

Current research about quantum healing addresses how individuals can achieve a deeper connection with the intelligence of this source design and with its capacity to naturally repair the body. Highly consistent with somatic art therapy, the quantum model assumes that consciousness is central to any disease and any healing journey (Goswami, 2013). As with Hamel's approach, this model looks at how our mind and our inner imagery affect the physical body, before its material form. In this regard, Hamel also uses consciousness as the key therapeutic driving force to access the healing frequencies and potentialities within the source design.

In order to understand the states of consciousness that actually support health and the outcome of our physical pain, we need to avoid any shortcuts that tend to oversimplify such a model. The large number of books that we currently see conferring magical virtues to positive thinking are good examples of this phenomenon. In addition to bringing a sense of guilt to individuals who are unable to manifest health through the power of thought alone, their use of quantum principles remains superficial. Unfortunately, picturing healing and visualizing that we are healthy in our mind's eye are not enough to make it a reality. Nor is it enough to avoid getting angry by exclusively trying to nurture positive vibes, hoping to experience a pain-free body and existence. These widespread misconceptions about the power of consciousness and the laws of manifestation are essentially reductive. The quantum model actually involves far more complex processes than just *concealing* our negative thoughts or imagining our ideal reality.

The elements required in the states of consciousness that enable, facilitate, or accelerate healing have nothing to do with *ordinary* thinking. Originating beyond our skull, these states of consciousness are not driven by the analytical mind that we tend to confine ourselves to. So, to understand the healing potentials inherent to our consciousness, it is crucial to focus, first and foremost, on the heart-brain.

## The heart as an intuitive brain

Contrary to popular belief, our head is not the leading conductor of our living experience. Indeed, the latest research in neurocardiology demonstrates that there is a second brain whose mechanisms prevail over cranial brain activity. Located in the heart, this brain has its own unique memory and is equipped with a nervous system that is separate from both brain hemispheres. Research conducted by the HeartMath[1] Institute enhances a critical breakthrough. The heart sends more information to the cranial brain than the other way around, playing a leading role in our body's regulating processes. These messages from the heart travel to the brain via ascending pathways in both the spinal column and along the vagal nerve, eventually reaching the medulla, the hypothalamus, the thalamus, the amygdala, and the cerebral cortex.[2] This amazing discovery shows that communication between the cranial brain and the heart-brain is far from being unidirectional, as we have long thought it was.

However, heart-brain states of consciousness are not organized in the same way as those originating from the cranial brain. They rely mostly on intuitive processes, in the sense that the realm of intellectual, linear, and analytical thinking specific to the logical mind is not involved. Unfortunately, throughout the evolution of the human species, we moved away from these states of consciousness, placing a wedge within our capacities for self-healing.

As an art therapist, I have great interest for heart-brain states of consciousness, as they are a key therapeutic driving force when it comes to helping individuals engage with their own healing processes. From an experiential perspective, the greatest advances made by my clients often occur precisely once they give up the reference points of their analytical and logical mind in favour of their intuitive intelligence. It is a highly effective gateway to access what Eckhart Tolle defines as a *no-mind gap,* which is a state of consciousness where the individual is *much more alert, more awake than in the mind-identified state* (2004, 19–20). In his book *The Power of Now* (2004), Tolle describes the mind as a wonderful tool when used properly. He emphasizes, however, that most of us are enslaved to the mind without even being aware of it, holding on to the mistaken belief that the mind is our whole Being. His best-known statement certainly is: 'You are not your mind'. Tolle sees the ability to generate *discontinuity in our mental stream* as a necessary state of consciousness to raise 'the vibrational frequency of the energy field that gives life to the physical body' (Tolle, 2004, 20).

In my art therapy studio, I often witness how the creative process is a concrete way of accessing discontinuity in the mental stream of consciousness as described by Tolle. To the untrained eye, the creative and intuitive processes generating a no-mind gap might seem absurd, fragmented, senseless, incoherent, esoteric, or even ineffective. However, experienced art therapists know how to tap into these genuine healing and transformative potentials. Contrary to popular belief and, despite its apparent discontinuity, our intuitive intelligence has its own architecture which is not framed by the linear algorithms specific to intellectual points of reference. One might be led to believe, wrongly so, that it is totally random and nonsignificant. Make no mistake about it. Intuitive intelligence is a vital *muscle* for any healing process, although it has a set of rules totally different from those of the rational and logical mind.

In my private practice, mind identification, as defined by Tolle, is often the main obstacle that my clients face as they try to enter the states of consciousness needed to resolve pain and symptoms responsible for physical and emotional suffering. In general, the modern human being is looking for answers in his head, even though this does not offer much relief. Cut off from parts of ourselves that are so essential, we somehow became illiterates of the heart-brain states of consciousness. In individual sessions, I am frequently called upon to rehabilitate one's capacity to simply *feel,* as clients have grown more and more disconnected from their body, their heart, and their presence. In many ways, their conscious mind is completely overinvested in automatic, involuntary, and compulsive thinking, replaying the same loop over and over again, with hypervigilance. Here, my work focuses on re-educating their awareness so that they can restore their connection to their heart and to their felt sense, almost like relearning to use atrophied muscles that were left inactive for too long.

Now that the heart-brain's significant role in regulating our bodies has been confirmed by neurocardiology research, it is appropriate to ask ourselves which therapeutic means should be preferred to maximize its healing potentials.

## Experiential method: somatic heart coherence. Restoring the connection with the overlooked brain

Owing to the primacy of the mind over the heart in our modern cultures, we might reach the conclusion that cutting ourselves off from the heart-brain is depriving us from an intelligence that is vital to our health. How can we possibly restore the lines of communication with this central organ? In my view, *somatic art therapy* provides a particularly interesting avenue in this regard. Therefore, I created an experiential method intended to foster a direct connection with heart-brain states of consciousness. I named this experiential method *somatic heart coherence*. My clinical intention is to specifically support one's ability to engage with the conscious source design and tap into its self-healing potentials.

Based on the *hands-on healing* method presented by Hamel in chapter 10, the individual begins illustrating his heart soma by focusing on the physical sensation felt in this powerful organ. This involves connecting with the felt sense and the body's somatic dimension as defined by Levine (2008). For instance, one might connect with a feeling of heaviness in the chest. This somatic aspect can also manifest itself as a tightness of the heart or a feeling that the organ is somehow enclosed within a sealed armour. You might even connect with a barely perceptible vibration or an abstract fear that initiates thoracic constrictions. Here, it is appropriate to use a large piece of paper to amplify the person's connection with her somatic sensations. Getting away from any stereotypical imagery of the heart is also important, as we want the individuals to tap into their own unique visual language, one that is rooted in the body's subjective felt sense.

Once this step is completed, engaging in *somatic listening* (Rinfret, 2000) with the image will be necessary to carve out the existential message delivered by the heart and the body. This part of the experiential method requires us to tap into the states of consciousness available outside of the marked-out paths of rational thinking. In this regard, the creative process has already initiated a shift towards discontinuity in the mind stream. At this point, maintaining the connection with the physical sensation present in the heart is important, even if the drawing process is over. This will help the person to grasp the existential message as Hamel suggests. A healing colour can be applied only once that message has been identified.

To illustrate how to use the physical heart as a portal of connection to the quantum design and its intrinsic healing potentials, here is a case study of an individual who experienced my *somatic heart coherence* method.

### Case study: The reunification

Emily (fictitious name) is an art therapy student in her thirties, attending an intensive course that I teach on *somatic art therapy* at the Université du Québec en Abitibi-Témiscamingue (Québec, Canada). In previous art therapy exercises before I introduced the *somatic heart coherence* experiential method, she revealed a strong tendency to turn her anger back onto herself.

Among the significant images drawn previously, she created a full-sized figure that accurately illustrates retroflection of her anger. In this representation of her silhouette, we can see her body's contours covered with lacerations that look like self-mutilating scars left by a razor blade. This image reveals to us the violent feelings inside Emily's body. While sharing her experience with me, she expressed feeling disconnected from her body, even feeling at times as if it did not belong to her. Getting in touch with her proprioceptive input felt

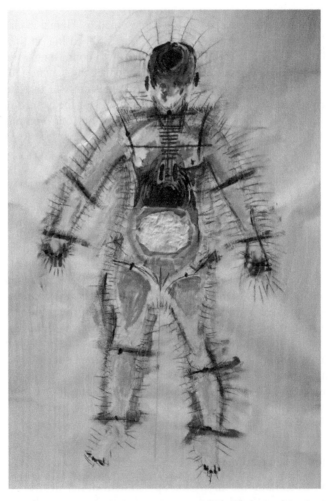

*Figure 9.1* Emily's silhouette, before the introduction of *somatic heart coherence*, 5 feet x 7 feet (152 cm x 215 cm), chalk pastels and gouache.

painful, and any classroom activity intended to focus on soma made her aware of how tense, invaded, and even fragmented she was when it comes to her body schema. She mentioned experiencing episodes of depersonalization before, where she no longer knew who she was and felt alien to herself. She also shared with me having recurring suicidal thoughts and cyclical depression for several years. The process that she engaged in during my class helped her to become more aware of how difficult taking care of herself was, as she began noticing her self-destructive patterns. To quote her exact words, her healing intention through this process was to *let go of her tendency to harm herself.*

Following a guided meditation designed to help my students get in touch with their heart soma, everyone was invited to move over to a large sheet of white paper attached to the wall and to visually lay down their feelings. Shyly, Emily started to give shape to the subjective sensation in her chest. She used wooden pencils on a huge 5-feet x 5-feet piece of paper, intensely sketching the organ's muscular tissues. She also attempted to depict the emotions and sensations entrenched in these fibers. Even though she had been drawing for more than 45 minutes, her lines and shapes were so faint that her sketch was barely visible. I had to look quite closely at the paper to see the illustration that she had created.

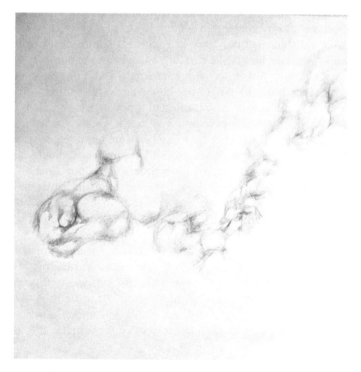

*Figure 9.2* Emily's representation of the heart soma (part one), 5 feet x 5 feet, 152 cm x 152 cm, color pencils.

Taking a step back from the image, Emily expressed surprise at how much her heart felt withdrawn and enclosed. However, while creating it, she felt as if she was using a lot of space. She was almost tearful as she became aware of this. While her heart was tiny and seemed almost transparent in the middle of a white sea of empty space, it had *finally* appeared. She then expressed feeling a deep sense of gratitude towards herself. With great emotion, she said *I may be small, but I am present.* At this point, getting in touch with her heart soma allowed her to achieve broader awareness about something that indeed had eluded her: *It feels like I never could exist.* The somatic aspect of her heart had opened the gate to her intuitive intelligence. Through that, Emily became aware of how she had lived disconnected from her body, her heart, and her whole Being. This was her existential message.

At this point, her facial expression had drastically changed, and her body was shedding, one layer at a time, the overwhelming heaviness felt throughout the intensive week. While she had been self-harming at the beginning of the class, she now was in the process of opening up to something much broader than ordinary consciousness. As a witness of her transformation, I can honestly say it felt as if Emily was giving birth to herself through the creative process.

Following that first step, the whole group was invited to carry on the experiential method by applying a healing color, as suggested by Hamel in chapter 10. Still shaken, Emily moved back to her drawing to further the reunification with her heart. She carefully mixed various paints to create a soft turquoise color. Great softness emanated from this shade of color specifically blended to take care of her little heart. This softness contrasted with the visual indicators of retroflected anger that she had created throughout the week. With care and gentleness, Emily started applying paint around her heart, with her bare hands. Using her fingers to make the pigment glide over the paper, it almost felt like she was applying ointment onto the image. In doing so, an outward expansion movement lovingly arose. Her meaningful gestures became sacred, and the ritual unfolding between Emily and her heart made us aware that this was an extremely precious and powerful moment. Witnessing her deep connection with her image makes it very clear that *art is a prayer*, in other words, a transcendent experience as defined by Zinker (2006, 16). To me, sacredness is a substrate of the heart-brain states of consciousness. Through it, we leave behind our everyday *habitual and functional* consciousness to dive in to the mystical and invisible dimension within oneself. By ritually stroking the image with care, intention, and presence, Emily was immersed in a deeply significant experience that allowed her to resolve the somatic effects of her retroflected anger.

Soft turquoise colored ripples gradually took shape around Emily's sheer heart, somehow reproducing the structure of a cosmic vortex. Her gestures were calming, and her whole body was engaged in the experience.

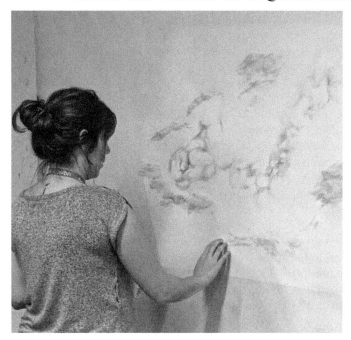

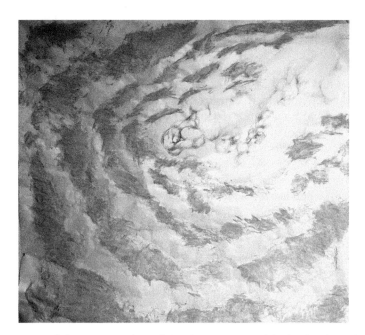

*Figure 9.3* Emily's representation of her heart soma, with the *hands-on healing* method (part two), 5 feet x 5 feet (152 cm x 152 cm), color pencils and gouache. On the bottom: the completed image, 5 feet x 5 feet (152 cm x 152 cm), colour pencils and gouache.

By filling in the initially vacant space around the heart with increasing confidence, Emily realized that this *empty* space was hers and that she had the right to step into it. She portrayed her felt sense as energy waves gently and harmoniously emerging from her heart, settling into her whole body. Some sort of somatic coherence began to manifest itself as Emily's creative process unfolded, leading her to integrate her physical, cognitive, emotional, and spiritual dimensions into one unified whole. She was leaving her fragmented self behind. Looking at her image with great love and compassion, Emily shared that she *no longer felt alone*. It was as if she had witnessed a reunification between the scattered parts of herself.

After applying the healing colour, Emily's energy was totally transformed. Tears of joy were rolling down her cheeks, and deep emotions were running through her whole Being as she talked about her image. She was quite surprised by her own overwhelming enthusiasm, which was a true departure from her depressed mood throughout the week. Emily expressed having deep feelings of love for herself for the first time in her life. She felt that she had offered herself a *declaration of love*, saying that she had finally *found Emily*. These words reflect how she returned to her heart and to her body just like we come back home after being away for a long time. On a somatic level, she went through a radical transformation, as the quality of her presence was enhanced and life was again flowing through her. The stiffness in Emily's body went away, allowing for a state of openness both to herself and to others. That genuine attitude was not initially present. We could sense her breath reaching deeper as her chest was opening up. She now embodied herself in a more relaxed and grounded way as joy and relief radiated from her facial expression. She shared her experience in a vibrant way, and her depressed mood throughout the process had vanished. Emily's mortifying relationship with her body had alchemized into self-love. She also had the physical sensation of being fully embodied, feeling like she was taking up a lot of space compared with the beginning of her journey. She now felt a powerful surge of energy coming from her heart and providing great relief from the retroflected anger that she had worked on throughout the class. She no longer wanted to harm herself, which was a very touching moment for those of us witnessing her journey.

In that cathartic moment of somatic coherence, Emily reclaimed the body that she had become alienated from. However, that deep reunification goes far beyond the simple *physical* dimension. Emily's heart, body and mind were no longer fragmented. Experiencing great clarity and a sense of being held by something greater than herself, she shared these words with emotion: 'I am no longer alone, I am here, *with* myself'. Art therapist Anne-Marie Jobin states that: 'Along with meditation or relaxation, the act of creation has the potential to generate a connection with something bigger than us, if we only know how to surrender to the process' (Jobin, 2013, 35) (Free translation). This enhanced contact, which is described in Jobin's book *Créez la vie qui vous ressemble* (2013), can readily be compared with source design consciousness.

Looking at my student's journey, we quickly understand that the theoretical slideshow presentations that I gave in class are far from being responsible for that transformation! Rooted in heart-felt sense, it is the power of the experiential process that allowed Emily to stop identifying with her mind and reconnect in a loving way with her heart-brain. The energy that she was channeling while being acutely present to herself goes far beyond the states of consciousness of the ordinary ego. Clearly, Emily was able to tap into the states of consciousness necessary to access the quantum dimension, and it stands to reason that her transformation could not have occurred by verbal therapy alone.

## The quantum power of self-love

A number of studies confirm the role and the importance of love to maintain our health (Lipton, 2016). For instance, it has been demonstrated by neuroscientist James Coan that the levels of pain and anxiety in an individual will significantly be reduced when offered the possibility to hold hands with a loved one (Coan, Schaefer, and Davidson, cited in Lipton, 2016). This study also shows that the healthier and the stronger the bond is with that loved one, the less physical pain and fear will be present. Now, what about self-love and its self-healing powers? In my case study, Emily was able *to hold her own hand*, which offered a meaningful and healing experience. Feeling through her physical heart that she was 'there for herself' and no longer 'alone' greatly contributed to the psychosomatic breakthrough she experienced with the *somatic heart coherence* experiential method.

In truth, available science exploring the actual quantum and biological power of self-love is limited. Unfortunately, most research is still articulated around a paradigm of separation between body and soul without really looking into our own inherent restorative potentials. Anita Moorjani, the author of the best-selling book *Dying to be Me* (2014), offers a convincing testimony about the power of self-love on our soma, our body, and our cells. While at the end of her life with terminal cancer, Anita explains how she became filled with unconditional love for herself as, comatose, she was preparing to 'die'. In this near-death experience, she remembers entering a quantum and multidimensional space where she realized that she had always lived in fear of not being *enough*. As her consciousness expanded beyond her physical form, Anita understood that her quest for love and external validation had led her to 'violate' her own truth by seeking the acceptance of others. This vibrational space of infinite love in which she felt immersed allowed her to somehow initiate a 'reunification' with what Goswami defines as the Quantum Self (2013). Upon reconnecting with her *Essence* and her *Truth*, Anita also reconnected with the intelligence of the source design from which she had cut herself off over time. While her doctors informed her husband that she would not make it through the night, she chose to return into her physical body to give herself the love that she had been longing for her whole life. Here, we can easily draw a parallel with Emily, who also offered herself unconditional love during the art therapeutic experiential process.

Despite an aggressive lymphoma that she had battled for four years and the shutdown of all her organs, Moorjani came out of her coma. Within a few weeks, her body had completely regenerated itself, showing no trace of cancer whatsoever. While her consciousness transcended the cause of her disease, we cannot grasp nor explain this healing based on a materiality paradigm. Anita returned home completely healed and now shares, internationally, the lessons that she learned during her few *end-of-life* days.

While Moorjani experienced near-death in order to reclaim her self-love and heal, there is no need to go through such an experience to access the regeneration potentials available in the source design. The quantum space that provides a heightened state of presence and a deep sense of love can readily be accessed by the human body, right here on Earth! Emily's experience, and that of many individuals I guide daily, shows me that this space is fully accessible to us when we go beyond our usual and conditioned thought patterns.

However, I believe that most of us need to rediscover how to connect with the somatic coherence offered by the heart. In my opinion, the approach that Hamel presents in this book provides concrete avenues to achieve this goal as we explore soma through imagery. Most importantly, *somatic art therapy* gives us the opportunity to cultivate states of consciousness rooted in the intuitive intelligence required to access the quantum reality design.

## Understanding intuitive intelligence

The HeartMath Institute[3] looks closely at intuitive intelligence circuits and teaches people how to align with their healing potentials. You might already know this Institute for its contribution to the development of the heart coherence model based on the most recent breakthroughs in neurocardiology. As well as demonstrating how the heart-brain holistically regulates the body through the practice of gratitude, its research address three types of intuitive thinking in individuals.[4]

The first type of intuition is based on *implicit learning* that we acquired in the past and then forgot. It also refers to knowledge that we did not realize we had learned and somehow recorded without our conscious attention. Through this type of intuitive thinking, the cranial brain recognizes patterns from implicit memories based on our past experiences. It uses this database to solve new problems, without needing full analysis for decision-making. Its raw material is the past.

The second type of intuitive thinking refers to the *energetic sensitivity* of the nervous system, which detects electromagnetic signals from the environment and reacts to them in a subtle way. With this type of intuitive intelligence, people can detect, on a sensory level, the wavelengths issued by thoughts, emotions, and the environment through their body's soma. Certain people with highly developed sensitivity have the capacity to feel such vibrational and electromagnetic energy in all circumstances, whereas others can barely perceive it. A concrete example of energetic sensitivity to an overall heavy atmosphere is sometimes reflected by statements such as 'the tension was so thick you could cut it with a knife'. Invisible tensions between people can be energetically felt, even when there is no open and direct confrontation. Energetic sensitivity is quite common in children, as they do not go through the intellect to decode situations. Their nervous system instantaneously responds to the surrounding energetic matter.

*Non-local intuition* is of great interest to me and is the third type described by the Institute. This form of intuition is neither related to implicit past experiences nor to energetic sensitivity. Anchored in the ability to reach out for data that is *external* to us, its input does not come from our immediate environment but rather from the source design, as discussed above. As demonstrated by the HeartMath Institute research, the physical heart operates this non-local intuitive faculty rather than the cranial brain. What is of interest here is that this type of intuition connects us with information that transcends one's knowledge and personality.

To demonstrate how this type of intuitive intelligence works in regard to the source design, I would like to recount how it guided me to prevent a young girl's abduction by a prostitution network. Using my own personal experience as an example, I intend to illustrate the architecture of non-local intuition in our daily landscape.

My relationship with the type of intuitive thinking presented by the HeartMath Institute started occurring a few months before the actual event. Before the incident happened, I was inhabited by a brief, spontaneous but recurring image of a person so intoxicated that her own life was in danger. Having worked in the field of drug addiction and homelessness earlier in my career, I initially thought that this *image* surfaced randomly out of my counselling background. I did not understand why this image would flash in my mind, and I could not put a name on the intoxicated person's face nor associate it with any of my acquaintances.

Intrigued by that blurred vision that kept surging inside of me day after day, I began paying more attention to it. As I became more and more in contact with that peculiar *flash*, some sort of film automatically started unfolding inside of me; a film where I was playing a first responder role, so to speak. Without directing them, the images and somatic sensations were scrolling by exactly as if I was at the movies but inside of my own body. I felt calm, non-judgemental, and deeply empathic towards this person who had self-harmed through extreme substance abuse. As the film became clearer day after day, I could see myself trying to assist this person to ensure her safety. On my inner screen, I could see and feel that the person's life was in danger because of the high level of intoxication in her body. This was why my mind and my heart where trying to *rescue* her. But I also felt that I needed to protect this person from an impending external threat, owing to her extremely vulnerable state.

While my self-talk was trying to minimize the phenomenon by discrediting it, I still found myself rehearsing morning after morning what I would say to offer my assistance in such a situation. I would first ask the person to stand up, even though she was highly intoxicated. To assess the gravity of the situation, I would question which specific substance was used and how much was ingested. I would also ask whether this person would allow me to call for paramedics, and so on. I also saw myself pushing away people who were trying to take advantage of the situation. All this was going through my mind while I was blow-drying my hair, staring in the mirror, and wondering what it all meant! After rehearsing for many months, I had completely memorized my script, and my body felt strong and calm while embodying it. However, I still could not figure out what the point was!

Then one evening, I invited a friend downtown for a bite to eat. Departing from our usual routine, I suggested that we walk to get there. While wandering around chatting about everything and nothing, I saw from a distance, a young girl lying on a public bench, completely drunk. Highly intoxicated, her companion in his late teens was trying his best to keep her conscious. As soon as I saw her, I quickened my pace instinctively and ran towards the scene, leaving my friend behind without a second thought. Like in my rehearsals, I stepped into the first responder role that I had been practicing for months. I did not need time to think. Despite the urgency of the situation, I felt unwaveringly calm and grounded, which came as a surprise to both my friend and me.

While I was monitoring the young girl's vital signs and trying to keep her conscious until the paramedics arrived, a luxury car with tinted windows suddenly made a U-turn while driving past the scene. In both a suspect and puzzling way, two men in their early twenties got out of the car with confidence, offering to take the young girl to a hospital *for* us. At this point, I think it is worth mentioning that the young girl was in an alcohol-induced coma. She would come out of it for just a few seconds to throw up while I was struggling to keep her standing straight to prevent her from choking on her own vomit. She no longer had control over her body, as it was completely inanimate. My work experience in the field allowed me to understand that these guys were pimps. If my friend and I had arrived five minutes later, the young girl would have been kidnapped without any resistance on her part or on the part of her inebriated buddy. He was completely unable to protect her. These two men fortunately raced off when they found out emergency responders were on their way, which ensured that this young girl was safely transported to the hospital.

Now, one can easily understand that I do not have any *special powers*, but rather, an ability to connect with non-local intelligence as I faced such a difficult intervention. Just as Emily was able to connect with a matrix of consciousness far greater than herself through somatic art therapy, I believe that the same is true for the assistance given to that young girl. Without this ability to connect with my inner imagery and listen to the non-local intuition language of the heart, perhaps I would never have noticed that distraught girl in the distance. Or I might have frozen owing to the intensity of that moment, finding myself unable to act.

On both a small and a large scale, the non-local intelligence presented by the HeartMath Institute[5] is crucial for our health and our global balance. However, on a collective level, its potentials tend to be minimized or turned into mere esoteric and paranormal phenomena. Accessing non-local intuition is in fact consistent with Goswami's definition of *a quantum leap in consciousness* (2013). It refers to our consciousness's ability to make non-local connections with all things beyond time and space, leaving our personality and ego-based consciousness behind. The action of stepping into an *extraordinary* state of presence is therefore what we can refer to as a quantum leap. Consciousness, which is experienced as plural and fragmented, and which occurs in several *times* and *individuals,* then shifts to a unique mode. This is what Goswami refers to as unity consciousness (2013).

## Conclusion

Upon contact with her art therapy imagery, it is through unity consciousness that Emily was able to feel that she was no longer *alone*. It is again based on this unity consciousness that Moorjani experienced quantum healing of her terminally ill cancer without any external treatments. It is also through that same unity consciousness that I was able to be a proper channel, in the right place at the right time, to become 'one' with the right sequence of actions.

According to Goswami (2013), quantum physics clearly demonstrates that we are given the choice between disease and healing. However, it is important to master the quantum leap process towards unity consciousness in order to make this kind of *choice*. Many of us are already able to perform such leaps at different times of our lives, without really understanding how we succeed at it. Spontaneous recovery and placebo effects are great examples of these phenomena where consciousness alone can transform matter (Lipton, 2016). However, it is now clear that we cannot reach and alter our body's source design through ordinary thinking. That is why enhancing our ability to be present to the heart-brain is required. *Somatic art therapy* is a reliable approach in this regard, as it opens a window of discontinuity in our mental stream, thereby amplifying our capacity to tap into the states of consciousness that hold knowledge from non-local intelligence.

In the art therapy studio, I observe people transition towards unity consciousness when they start feeling clueless about their artwork. In those moments of confusion, they are actually leaving behind the known and redundant pathways of earlier conditioning to tap into heart-brain states of consciousness. When people do not control or understand rationally what is happening on their sheet of paper, they begin to connect with channels of non-local knowledge. That is precisely when they are presented with the opportunity to make a quantum leap in consciousness. Based on my experience, I know that my client, in this very moment, is on the brink of achieving a form of awareness that will dramatically transform her or his connection to her or his body, soma, and emotions. If we successfully remain focused in this field of consciousness, the person will connect directly with source design and its inherent self-healing potentials.

However, reconnecting with the heart-brain through *somatic art therapy* requires certain skills, and it is not uncommon for people who engage with my experiential method to initially experience a sense of inner emptiness, which is then reflected on paper. The creative process often allows them to realize they have cut off from their heart as a way to survive suffering. So, simply drawing one's heart is not enough for magic to happen. Counselling by a professional art therapist is critical to navigate through the vulnerable shifts that occur when one comes into contact with that void and soma. The therapist's ability to hold the required *temenos* (Duschastel, 2012) is essential for people to become familiar with the inner land that was left deserted as a result of deep suffering. Therefore, knowing how to 'provide a safe, confidential and protected space to explore the deepest and most sacred parts in each of us' (Duchastel, 2012, 32) (free translation) is a key element of the method presented here. Contacting the heart soma without the power of *presence* and *temenos* would be technical and profane. This would keep the client within the continuum of ordinary consciousness. To conclude, restoring *somatic heart coherence* through art therapy seems to be an effective way of reducing the deeply entrenched separation between body, heart, mind, and source design, both individually and collectively. However, beyond the high healing potentials offered by both the quantum model and *somatic art therapy*, it is their use of consciousness as a key therapeutic driving force that makes them suitable approaches to rightly guide us toward the origins of our diseases.

## Notes

1 www.heartmath.org/research/science-of-the-heart/heart-brain-communication, accessed August 6, 2020.
2 www.heartmath.org/research/science-of-the-heart/heart-brain-communication/, accessed August 6, 2020.

3  www.heartmath.org/research/science-of-the-heart/heart-brain-communication/ accessed August 6, 2020.
4  www.heartmath.org/research/science-of-the-heart/intuition-research/, accessed August 6, 2020.
5  www.heartmath.org/research/science-of-the-heart/intuition-research/, accessed August 6, 2020.

# Part IV
# Somatic Art Therapy Applications

# 10 Somatic Art Therapy Intervention Methods for Chronic Pain

*Johanne Hamel*

The art process therapy approach underlies all somatic art therapy principles and techniques, especially the hands-on healing method in this chapter. Rhinehart and Engelhorn's (1982) art process therapy approach was born from the addition of pre-images to the therapeutic process, i.e. taking into consideration lines, shapes, and colors as drawn by the client. The authors believe that finished images are just a part of the client's overall visual expression, as they have noticed that images can take a whole new perspective after in-depth exploration of the meaning of lines, shapes, and colours by the client and the art therapist.

This chapter will cover four different methods that I recommend to work on chronic or acute pain: the 'four-quadrants' method, hands-on healing, small silhouette drawing, and life-size silhouette. But as any art therapeutic exercise can be used as somatic art therapy if the drawing or painting relates to the inner body sensation or *soma*, I will also introduce *art process therapy* as a way to work with any soma exercise.

## The four-quadrants method

I created the four-quadrants method in 1997, taking inspiration from Achterberg (1985), Siegel (1994), and McNiff (1992), among others. Appendix C details the instructions for this exercise when used in a group where participants draw a giant mandala on a large 5-feet x 8-feet (1.5 m x 2.5 m) paper format. For examples of giant mandalas, see pages 107 and 110. In the following assignment examples, the four drawings are rather successively made on 18-inch x 24-inch (45 cm x 60 cm) paper sheets.

*First drawing*: The instruction is to draw a current or often present physical pain, focusing specifically on the painful *sensation*.

*Second drawing*: The instruction is to go back in time until a similar sensation was felt for the very first time and to figuratively represent the events or what the person felt like at the time. If no memory becomes available, the person draws the kind of situations in which this pain will come up.

*Third drawing*: The instruction given here is to draw again the contour of the same specific part of the body the person is working on, but this time, the person draws how that part would look like visually if the pain was totally gone, and if it would feel entirely good and even pleasurable.

*Fourth drawing*: For the last drawing, the instruction is to represent the transition between the first drawing (pain) and the third one (healing), either by borrowing visual features from the images drawn in both or by representing repressed feelings in the situation depicted in the second drawing.

The effect of this four-steps approach is to grasp the existential message of a pain (quadrant 1), to understand where the pain originates from (quadrant 2), to acknowledge what is possible (quadrant 4) and to understand how healing can be achieved (quadrant 3). Be aware that quadrant 4 is drawn before quadrant 3. Several case studies based on this method are presented in chapter 11.

## Hands-on healing

I further expanded the following method that was first taught to me by Rhinehart and Engelhorn (1984)[1]. The different steps are as follows:

### *Relaxation*

First, relax and identify a somatic sensation to work on. Focus on your breath without trying to alter it. Leave behind any concerns one by one, and tell yourself that you will take care of them later. Then focus on the sensations in your body. Identify one tension or discomfort. Do not try to alter the discomfort unless you feel uncomfortable because of your physical position, in which case moving a little should be enough to get more comfortable. Feel the discomfort, pain or sensation in its specificity to the greatest extent possible, basically to have a taste of it in some way.

### *Drawing*

This step involves drawing the tension or discomfort using lines, shapes or colors describing as closely as possible the somatic sensation as felt. Use oil pastels or felt-tip pen, so that the color can be later covered with another wet medium for hands-on healing.

### *Dialogue*

Then initiate a dialogue with the discomfort by reproducing and enhancing lines, shapes, and colors on paper. If lines could talk, for example, what would they say? Replicate them on several sheets of paper, until their meaning becomes clear. Proceed the same way with colors: what feelings, memories, emotions, or insights do they give rise to within you? With forms, expand them by drawing only their contour in a larger way. Then imagine you are seeing what is *inside* the form, drawing any kind of images coming to your mind. Again, what feelings, memories, emotions, insights do those images give rise to within you? When the psychological meaning of the discomfort is clear to you, go to the next step. This meaning is important to understand, otherwise the healing color that you will apply later on will only artificially hide the discomfort.

### *Meditation with a healing color*

The healing color is personal, it needs to feel soothing to you at that precise moment and for that sensation. Do not hesitate to mix several colors to get exactly the right shade. As an example, too dark pink or green might no longer be felt as soothing, once applied to a drawing about tension. Decide on a healing color and use it with the drawing on tension made in step #2, according to one of the following:

- Apply this color around the illustrated pain, tension or discomfort;
- Use finger paint to cover the illustrated pain, tension or discomfort for *hands-on healing*; or
- Cover the illustrated pain, tension or discomfort with silk paper or painted cotton wool of the healing color…

If you chose to work on a pleasant sensation rather than on a tension or discomfort, just enhance it on the sheet of paper by reproducing it in an even bigger way, or using a more flowing medium or with more vibrant colours, for instance. And see what happens to you by doing so.

## Small silhouette drawing

Here, you are invited to draw the contours of a silhouette on a 18-inch x 24-inch (45 cm x 60 cm) sheet of paper, then to draw your body sensation within that shape. Anne-Marie Jobin proposes her own version to work on injuries, pains and diseases:

> Draw two silhouettes, one of which represents the front of the body and the other one, the back. Pick up four different colors to illustrate the following: comfort, discomfort, acute tension, disease. Color the silhouettes according to these four sensations. Add all the words and phrases that come to you while looking at your drawing, then take note of your thoughts.

(2002, p. 74)

I have personally used this silhouette exercise to work on acute pain or discomfort related to chemotherapy and radiotherapy. Indeed, as art therapy allows visualization on paper, I found out that participating in one's own treatment in this way is possible and helps to reduce the adverse effects of radiotherapy or chemotherapy. I worked with clients whose nausea and fatigue were considerably reduced by making drawings before and after chemotherapy treatments. They represented the chemotherapy drugs passing through their bodies producing beneficial effects and drew the chemicals that need not be kept or that could damage healthy cells passing out of their bodies. The visualization of radiotherapy rays filling the body as a regenerating golden light has been used successfully for the purpose of reducing fears of such treatment, better accepting it, as well as reducing its adverse effects, such as fatigue.

## Life-size silhouette

You can also ask your art therapist to draw the contours of your actual figure on a large sheet of paper by tracing them around your body. Then, draw the sensation in each part of your body inside the traced silhouette. I usually suggest doing it for the front of the body, but this can also be done with the back of the body. In itself, this exercise will give you a lot of information about the condition of your entire body, as well as about the discomfort or painful sensations throughout your body. It will also provide information about real or symbolic connections between your different ailments. Then you might want to explore the different areas of your body more specifically, using the previously proposed approaches.

## Art process therapy

Any art therapy exercise can become *somatic*, as long as we focus on the inner sensation or *soma*. In these cases, we will mostly use the *art process therapy* approach (see chapter 1).

The *art process therapy* approach underlies all somatic art therapy principles and techniques, especially the hands-on healing method in this chapter. For Rhinehart and Engelhorn (1982), the *art process therapy* approach was born from the addition of pre-images to the therapeutic process, i.e. taking into consideration lines, shapes, and colours as drawn by the client. The authors believe that finished images are just a part of the client's overall visual expression; they noticed that images can take on a whole new perspective after in-depth exploration of the meaning of lines, shapes, and colours by the client and the art therapist. The *art process therapy* approach can either be used in a single therapy session or a long-term intervention.

Duchastel (2005) uses the *art process therapy* approach as follows when working on *soma*:

'Sometimes, the individual needs only to become aware of what is happening in his body to cause the emergence of a significant emotion or memory. Simple questions like "What's going on with your jaw? What would your restless foot say if it could speak? or What is the red patch in your neck trying to tell you?" allow the individual to engage in a revealing dialogue with these parts of himself. (…) We often find that one fails to recognize the emotion trying to come out. The individual will complain, for example, about a knot in his throat, chest tightness, solar plexus burning, tightness in the abdomen or knots in the back. In this case, the art therapist will suggest a drawing or a three-dimensional representation of the discomfort. In doing so, a prolonged contact with the body sensation is promoted and quite often, answers or new avenues to explore will emerge. When the individual finds the meaning of his discomfort, most of the time it has already disappeared or at least lost intensity.

(Duchastel, 2005, 177) (free translation)

## Note

1  Rhinehart, L. & Engelhorn, P. (1984). 'The full rainbow – Symbol of individuation'. *The Arts in Psychotherapy, 11*, 7–43.

# 11 'Four-quadrants' Method Case Studies

*Johanne Hamel*

Described in the previous chapter, this method is quite effective and can help to understand the meaning of physical discomfort; it can also alleviate chronic pain and even sometimes eliminate it permanently. Several examples are provided for the purpose of giving an idea of the range of impacts possibly obtained. All of the examples reported here are from individuals who completed the exercise at the *somatic art therapy workshop* or in connection with it.

First, I have a word of advice. Do you intend to experience this exercise by yourself? I do not recommend it, unless you have many years of experience working on yourself and learned about your significant personal issues. Even in this case, it is likely that you will come out with new information about yourself. This exercise can raise very intense emotions and bring up past traumatic experiences. If you want to do this all by yourself, please use dry media (felt pens, oil pastels, chalk pastels) and find a friend to accompany you. Consulting an art therapist to do this exercise, ideally a professional trained in the *art process therapy* approach, can prove essential, given the substantial potential effects of this exercise on the psyche and the soma.

Are you a psychotherapist or helping relationship professional, but not trained in art therapy? I do not recommend using this method on your clients. As mentioned above, intense emotions and traumatic experiences could be raised, and dealing with them through art could give you a hard time. Of course, you know what to do verbally with intense emotions, but this exercise will have raised images needing closure *through* images. Knowledge of the psychological impact of art media and know-how in terms of the art therapeutic process are required. If you were only doing verbal closure, the images could haunt your clients for a long time.

The following are five case studies using the 'four-quadrants' method; the process required to create either four 18-inch x 24-inch (45 cm x 60 cm) drawings (case study A) or a giant mandala (case studies B, C, D, E). To understand the following explanations, please remember that the third drawing of the giant mandala must be done within quadrant #4 and the fourth drawing within quadrant #3. For these case studies, I mostly chose the client's own words to describe their experience.

# Case study A

### Chronic pain in uterus

This first case study focuses on chronic pain associated with a traumatic situation.[1] My client is 39 years old and is attending a group art therapy weekend. She suffers from adhesions to the uterus, the colon, the intestine, the bone mass, and the muscle mass in this area of the body. These have often caused painful menstruation and constipation, as well as near-constant abdominal pains since the age of 15–16, with lull periods. She had three ectopic pregnancies in nine years; two of them were six months apart, and she had surgery for both. Two years ago, a third ectopic pregnancy was treated with methotrexate. Following this third pregnancy, she underwent tubal ligation. This client was sexually abused during childhood, of which she was fully aware, and she has worked on this several times in various psychotherapeutic contexts. I saw her a few times in a group, and a trusting relationship was already established.

The client was invited to experiment the four-quadrants exercise. The purpose was to work on physical wellness, trying to identify the images underlying physical pain, so as to better transform them.

### First drawing, quadrant 1: The painful sensation (see Figure 11.1)

The client was instructed to draw a current or often present physical pain, focusing specifically on the painful sensation. She chose to work on the pain in her abdomen. Figure 11.1 indicates a black hand strongly adhering to a

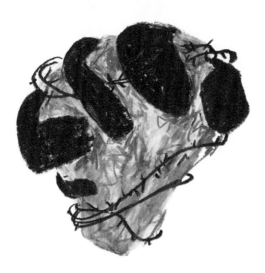

*Figure 11.1* (First drawing, quadrant #1) *The pain.* 18 inches x 24 inches (45 cm x 60 cm). Oil pastels.

pink, blue, and white uterus surrounded by barbed wire. The image renders the idea and sensation of *adhesions* to the uterus. The client felt the pain at the very moment that she was drawing it, and it was particularly activated since she started menstruating.

### Second drawing, quadrant 2: The past origin of the pain (see Figure 11.2)

For this one, the client was instructed to go back in time until a similar sensation was felt for the very first time. She had no memory, but a recent dream about a threatening storm came back to her mind. She first drew a huge black spot on the right side to depict the storm, then a blue shape reminiscent of a phallic shape, at the centre. Memories arose in her mind all of a sudden: at the age of seven or eight, she accidentally impaled herself by falling from above on an old wooden fence; a piece of wood penetrated from the groin to the pelvic bone, a few inches from the vulva. She was extremely moved to find this memory and to understand that it was associated with her current pains.

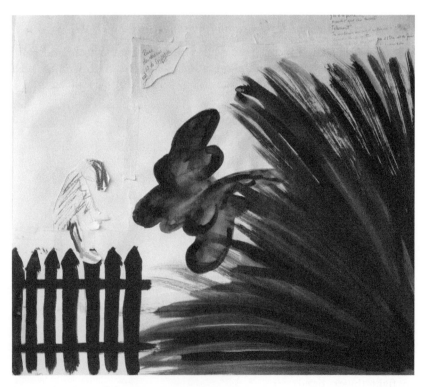

*Figure 11.2* (Second drawing, quadrant #2) *The past origin of the pain.* 18 inches x 24 inches (45 cm x 60 cm). Felt tips.

### Third drawing, quadrant #4: The healing (see Figure 11.3)

This time, she drew how it would feel if this part of her body healed completely. The client drew a rosy uterus which reminded her of pearls, sweetness, and flowers. With this drawing, a lot of sadness emerged, given that it seemed impossible that she would feel this good someday.

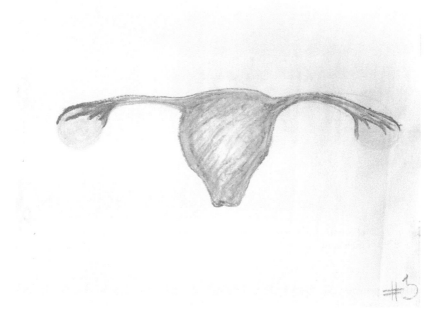

*Figure 11.3* (Third drawing, quadrant #4) *Healing.* 18 inches x 24 inches (45 cm x 60 cm). Oil pastels.

### Fourth drawing, quadrant #3: The transition (see Figure 11.4)

For the last drawing, the assignment was to represent the transition between the first drawing (pain) and the third one (healing) by borrowing visual features from the images drawn in both. The client drew the pink uterus once again. This time, it was held up in an open hand, spontaneously drawn in pale blue, whereas it was all black in the first drawing. To her, it meant to stop holding back her emotions and to allow herself to get in touch with tremendous sadness.

The shift to the blue colour revealed that a subjective image had been spontaneously transformed, which reflected a cognitive change in my client. Indeed, she realized that her adhesions were not an internal enemy to fight (black hand), nor a malfunctioning of some part of her body seeking to destroy another one, but an extreme protective response of the

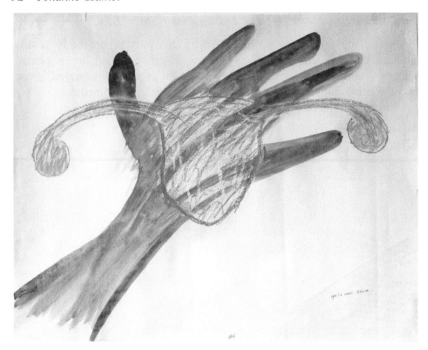

*Figure 11.4* (Fourth drawing, quadrant #3) *Transition to healing*. 18 inches x 24 inches (45 cm x 60 cm). Oil pastels and watercolours.

body spontaneously triggered by the *shock* from the accident on the fence. This caused a complete reversal of her subjective perception of the adhesions. When questioned, she said that after realizing this, it now seemed somewhat possible to feel really good someday. The next day, her menstrual pains had considerably decreased; she described them as less strong than what she had been experiencing for many years. Five weeks after the exercise, she said:

> 'After the art therapy weekend, I was menstruating again. Apart from a little pain for the first half-day, it went very well. Since my last pregnancy, I just had abnormal periods. The menstrual flow was brownish with clots, and now it has become steady and red. Furthermore, abdominal pain decreased in frequency and intensity. I still have cramps and constipation, but not on a permanent and constant basis. I am very pleased about that!'

My current hypothesis is that her abdominal pain will gradually decrease in frequency and intensity in the coming months, which was confirmed every time that I asked for feedback (after one, two, three years and so on).

# Case study B

## *Pain between the shoulder blades*

Following a group art therapy weekend, my client chose to work on a stubborn pain between her two shoulder blades. Her own words are used below to describe her experience with drawing on a giant mandala (free translation).

## *First drawing, quadrant #1: The painful sensation*

First, I had to focus here and now on a typical pain, a symptom, a familiar but disturbing sensation. Going through the various sensations in my body in a state of relaxation, I focused on the stubborn pain between my two shoulder blades. This insistent pain that radiated forward kept coming back, especially after meals, and it was aching intensely now.

In the first quadrant, I drew and painted what looked like a bird's head, followed by the sensation of weight within my shoulder blades, a sensation that turned into double locks; that sensation had already emerged during the intensive week and was now coming back. It was rather brown and not very attractive. The lines were for the most part curved and reversed. I went over and over these lines several times, almost in a trance-like state (see Figure 11.5).

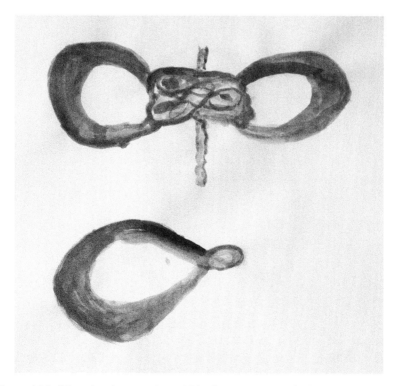

*Figure 11.5* (First drawing, quadrant #1) *The sensation.* 18 inches x 24 inches (45 cm x 60 cm). Tempera. (Reproduction).

I felt a rush of warmth to the face, while at the same time, I was moved to tears. It felt like sorrow, but I did not know what was really going on. Staying with that sensation, I continued to explore it.

### Second drawing, quadrant #2: The past origin of the pain

For the second quadrant, I had to go back to the past (see Figure 11.6). I was trying to remember the very first time that I had had this sensation, such a sense of discomfort. Nothing came back, and no image emerged spontaneously. Unable to find a way out of this impasse, I chose to initiate a dialogue with the double locks. Being confronted with my imagination led me to make a scribble in quadrant #2. The lines representing the bird with the letter 'M' at the tip of its beak were drawn in blue, and the two characters above in yellow.

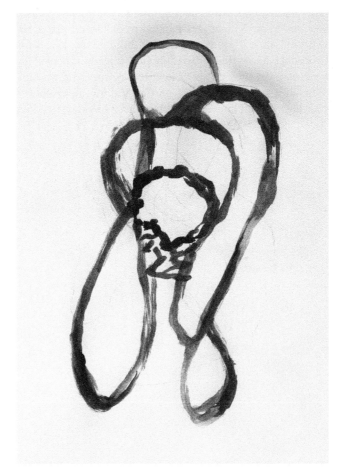

*Figure 11.6* (Second drawing, quadrant #2) *The past experience.* 18 inches x 24 inches (45 cm x 60 cm). Tempera. (Reproduction).

What came out of it left me speechless, pretty much like the bird. Now, the bird's beak was nailed, with an 'M' at its tip. The emerging image suggested a connection between my name because of the letter 'M'. Suddenly, I remembered asking my mother who had chosen my name. My father had named me after the wife of the local country store owner, with whom he was good friends. I do not know if my father also shared a friendship with this lady! My mother would have opted for another name, which is my middle name on my birth certificate. Yet the name M ......... was not my mother's choice; she often let my father decide without a word, repressing her feelings. As for me, I felt helpless and caught in the middle of these two yellow figures around me in the drawing. Feeling both my helplessness and my mother's grief, I was moved to tears and sobbed. Even my dog, lying on the floor far from me, suddenly jumped on the sofa to come and console me. He came up to me and licked my cheeks! It seems as if I cried a river for having felt caught up in the middle of my parents, helpless, and I also cried for the sadness that I shared with my mother.

### Third drawing, quadrant #4: The healing

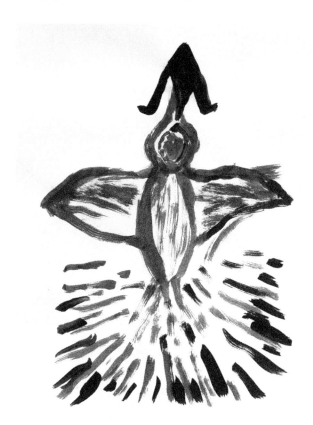

*Figure 11.7* (Third drawing, quadrant #4) *Healing of shoulder blades.* 18 inches x 24 inches (45 x 60 cm). Tempera. (Reproduction).

The third drawing in quadrant #4, the one for healing, was about how this part of my body would feel if it were completely healed. Feeling happy, I painted how I felt. I was as light as a bird that had just taken flight and was singing my name starting with an 'M', with strength and courage (red colour). Powerlessness gave way to strength, to the courage to be myself. Initially with only a head, the bird was now complete and light, just as I felt (see Figure 11.7).

### Fourth drawing, quadrant #3: The transition

As for the third quadrant, I was asked to draw the transition between the first quadrant (pain expressed through the felt sensation) and the last one (healing), while preserving visual elements of both (see Figure 11.8). I painted the locks that opened and the energy that circulated along my spine; green and yellow colours have replaced the initial brown one. While the bird still had just a head, he was more joyful and yellow; its beak was open with a big 'M' in front of him, and he was ready to sing my name.

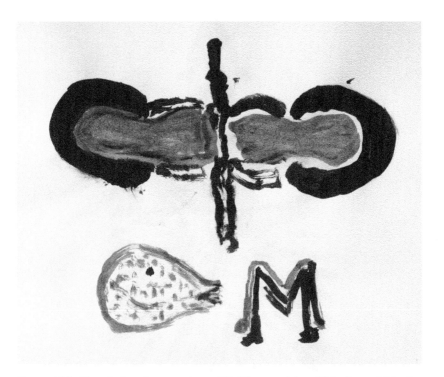

*Figure 11.8* (Fourth drawing, quadrant #3) *The transition.* 18 inches x 24 inches (45 cm x 60 cm). Tempera. (Reproduction).

While expressing my pain, it felt like the weight between my two shoulder blades was declining, and the lock was opening. After the exercise, I felt so clear and so good. Freed from this weight, I was feeling very light and surprised by such a discovery. I felt liberated, and I was breathing much better. I have been freed from this discomfort since then. I am quite proud of this, given that there was no need for pills or medication, as the change resulted from becoming aware of some childhood experiences affecting me. Even though these issues did not belong to me, I experienced them, and they marked my body. Discovering this came as a surprise. Through a lot a crying and tears, I felt the lock break apart. My sense of discomfort and the emotions of pain and helplessness stopped. I am so relieved! I never cease to be amazed by the power of the imaginary and where it leads me to.

## Case study C

### *A story about weight gain*

My 47-year-old client attended a *somatic art therapy* workshop for a week. She resumed the four-quadrants exercise at home after the workshop. The work she relates here is about her weight gain (free translation).

### *First drawing, quadrant #1: The painful sensation (see Figure 11.9)*

First, I sat down and took time to focus. I chose to sit on a bench for the first drawing which was about the sensation here and now (see Figure 11.9). I

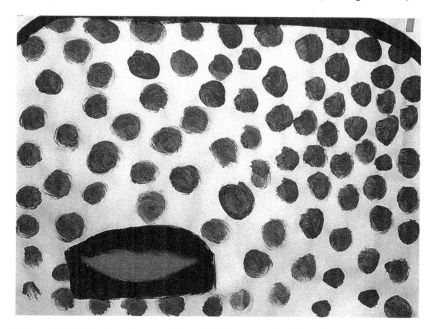

*Figure 11.9* (First drawing, quadrant #1) *Drawing the discomfort.* 18 inches x 24 inches (45 cm x 60 cm). Tempera.

wanted to work on my weight gain. I felt that the fat was gray (black for darkness and white for light). On the top right corner, I started tracing small concentric spheres moving from the outside to the inside, and I filled the whole paper sheet, progressing to the left (and to my past). As I was covering the sheet with drawings, I started feeling a pain between my shoulder blades. I always feel this pain when I am angry.

Then I felt that there was something vulnerable to protect; it was red, and when I set the brush on the paper, a mouth appeared and the following words emerged inside of me: 'As I am afraid of words and of other people's words, I am hiding behind fat to ward off the blows'. This image allowed me to acknowledge how I felt. In acknowledging this as a real experience, I understood what was going on inside of me. So in the first drawing, I discovered a connection between fat and unspoken words (mine and others'). I could see the fat in my body, imagine it, and put some distance with it: it's not my fat, it's only fat and I can draw it, gradually learning to distance myself from it.

### Second drawing, quadrant #2: The past origin of the pain (see Figure 11.10)

For the second drawing, a return to the past (see Figure 11.10), I sat on the floor like a 10-year-old little girl, the same age I was when I gained weight.

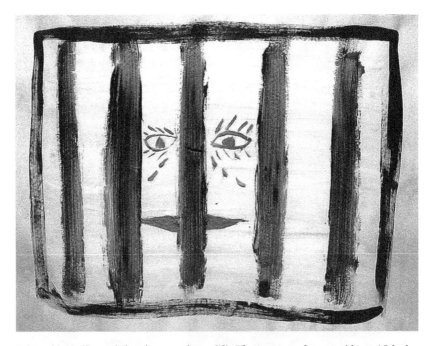

*Figure 11.10* (Second drawing, quadrant #2) *The imprisoned anger.* About 15 inches x 15 inches (about 38 cm x 38 cm). Tempera.

The fact is I was very thin until the age of ten, but after my father passed away, I quickly gained a lot of weight and never lost it. So I opted for this time of my life when I became overweight. The sensation that came up was related to feeling insignificant and unimportant. To illustrate this, I used white paint to trace horizontal lines, then I noticed a lower back pain. I added vertical black lines to represent my father's death; combined with the white colour, they became gray (like fat) and formed bars, then I drew myself in red behind bars. 'My anger is imprisoned and I strap myself into a sweet good girl straightjacket'. I also understood why my body got overweight: it was for defense and protection and for preserving my vulnerability. It might be that a potential threat around words was sensed in my body (my father died from throat cancer), and protection mechanisms were activated.

### Third drawing, quadrant #4: The healing (see Figure 11.11)

I drew myself standing upright, and surprisingly, I was turning my back. I felt open to space, the sea, my inner life, and life itself. I felt rooted in

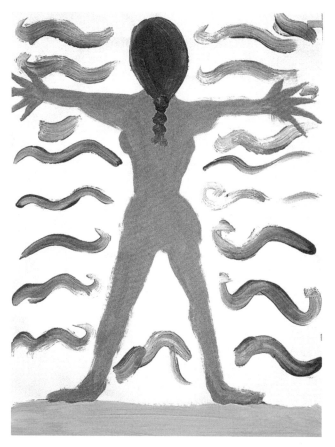

*Figure 11.11* (Third drawing, quadrant #4) *Healing.* About 15 inches x 15 inches (about 38 cm x 38 cm). Tempera.

green nature, and my hair was forming roots up in the sky. Pleased with the sensation of being in this healing space, I invested a lot into this drawing and took time to refine it.

### Fourth drawing, quadrant #3: The transition (see Figure 11.12)

The fourth drawing was about the transition to healing (see Figure 11.12). It required time for thinking, given that the previous ones seemed so different in terms of colors and content. Indeed, in the first drawing, my body was facing front, as I could actually see my mouth, while in the third one, I was turning my back. I represented myself from a side view, mouth wide open, spitting out fat molecules, with my nose, my eyes, my mouth, and my chin on the left side.

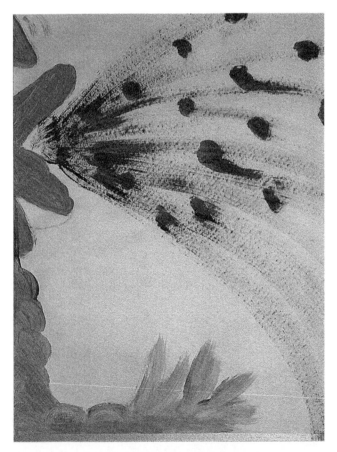

*Figure 11.12* (Fourth drawing, quadrant #3) *The transition.* About 15 inches x 15 inches (about 38 cm x 38 cm). Tempera.

The braided hair was helping me to take root. However, I noticed that my face was small in size on the paper, compared with the fat particles.

### About my process

Thinking back to my previous drawings, the feeling of transformative power I got from the healing one comes to mind; for a while, I was able to enjoy feelings of well-being, surrendering, daring to be who I am, opening myself to life, and letting life pulse inside of me. My body, through muscular tension (back pain) and its position during art creation (sitting, standing) was telling me a lot about the future journey to come to terms with my anger. I was also aware, when looking at my fourth drawing, that making such a change still felt risky, but I felt that I was on the path to healing (although small in size, my face is still there).

By making these drawings, I realized the full impact of images on my body. I felt muscular tension as I was drawing the body fat and even more tension over my whole back when drawing my past. My overweight associated with repressed emotions (anger), a pattern of self-deprecation, and how my body was trying to protect me. All this led me to believe that the transformation process was underway and that I would find new ways, other than being overweight, to ensure self-expression and self-protection. It is a matter of daring to be myself and taking my place verbally rather than physically.

During this experiential journey and through my drawings, I could feel what body fat meant in my life and envision new avenues for learning to express myself differently. What strikes me most in art therapy is that it is both rooted in reality and magical; it offers space and time to create possibilities and heal very old wounds.

Creation allows me to proceed at my own pace instead of matching the therapist's pace. What I draw on the paper sheet are images, images of my body and my world at the moment when I am ready to welcome them. Indeed, my subconscious can finally express itself and allow a new balance between the 'I' and the Self.

To conclude, I would add that through this last creation process, I got to know and to love myself better just the way I am, definitely not as sweet as before, but certainly more alive. Welcome to the Wolf in me that needs to howl!

## Case study D

### Spine disk herniation

The following example was reported by an art therapy student who was practicing the art therapist role. Her client was in her forties and had suffered a disk herniation for the last few months. Her own words are reported on the following pages (free translation).

### First drawing, quadrant #1: The painful sensation (see Figure 11.13)

For the first drawing, the client began by laughing and saying *I have nothing to work on,* while bending her arms and holding her palms face up. I invited her to repeat the same gesture, paying attention to her inner sensations. Here is what she wrote about the first drawing:

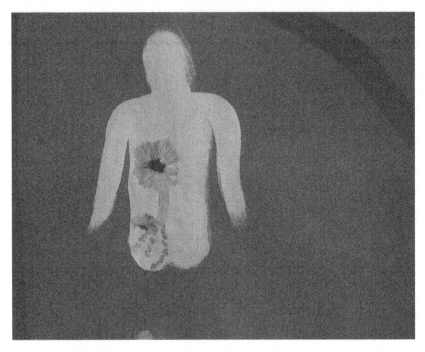

*Figure 11.13* (First drawing, quadrant #1) *The painful sensation.* About 15 inches x 15 inches (about 38 cm x 38 cm). Tempera.

When I started drawing, I could feel the pain at the level of the ninth vertebra. I drew the herniated disk while I was feeling a radiating sore point on the left side of my back. I was very afraid that the radiating pain in the leg would return as before.

She saw in her mind an image of a knife blade emerging from the pain at the ninth vertebra. At the same time, a childhood memory arose about a playmate who shoved her off a wall for no reason. She allowed herself to feel the blade in her back and noticed that it radiated down her lower left back, which she actually illustrated in the first drawing. It was a flesh-coloured figure seen from the back, without hands, legs, or support. The painful sensation was in red on the left side. The first quadrant allowed the client to feel her discomfort, to open up, and to pick an element to work on.

A sensation did emerge while at the beginning of the session she was not connected to the issue. The area with a radiating discomfort is consistent with a painful herniated disk from which she had recovered quite well, but which was still of concern to her. In short, attention and awareness enlightened the problem. At the same time, an image about the past was emerging. I realized that it would be important at this stage to temporarily set this memory aside and let the client draw it in quadrant #2 later on; this would allow her to focus entirely on the sensation in her body (i.e. the first quadrant).

### Second drawing, quadrant #2: The past origin of the pain (see Figure 11.14)

The client painted the childhood situation. She had nauseas and felt like being *caught in the middle of something* while drawing the wall on which a boy stands. There was a little girl on the grass. The situation brought back a strong feeling of misunderstanding: for no reason, an English-speaking

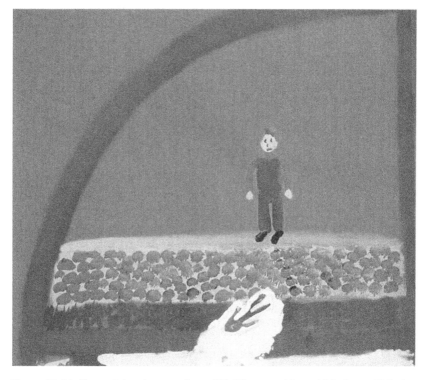

*Figure 11.14* (Second drawing, quadrant #2) *The past.* About 15 inches x 15 inches (about 38 cm x 38 cm). Tempera.

boy shoved her off a wall while they were both playing; she did not understand his language, but she was trying to avoid playing with the French-speaking children of the neighborhood, who were taller and always ended up hurting her. After the incident, he did not come to help. She saw the wall in the drawing as a turntable and the little girl as the needle '....crushed and pressured by the male character, unable to make it as long as he kept doing this to her' (her own words). The client released a lot of emotion during the process, and the sensation in her back decreased. In the second drawing, the most intense feeling was stated: a feeling of misunderstanding that, once identified, provided a catharsis with a decrease in physical discomfort.

### Third drawing, quadrant #4: The healing (see Figure 11.15)

The client represented the healing situation. Several characters, all the same size, naked and *untagged* (her own word), were playing with her. The

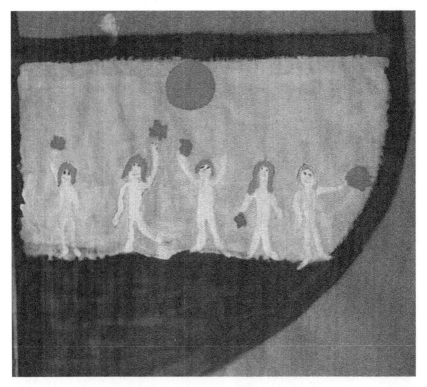

*Figure 11.15* (Third drawing, quadrant #4) *The healing.* About 15 inches x 15 inches (about 38 cm x 38 cm). Tempera.

second character from the left was her. I noticed that the legs, the ground and the hands had emerged. The colour of the injury was no longer there, but the wound's core shape was now inside the balloon that she was holding. It was a *sun-coloured energy* balloon. The client was aware that there was a sense of space and movement in the drawing as well of vulnerability (nudity). During the creation of this drawing, I observed that the client had faster, more fluid movements, as well as lateral movements of the head and twisting motions of the upper body; her movements though space were very different from the body stiffness and the 'frozen' movements shown in drawings #1 and #2. Obviously, the body was already undergoing some transformation. A liberating therapeutic effect was thus experienced in the body, following the cathartic expression of emotions in quadrant #2. Here, it is worth noting that my client spontaneously interpreted the instruction as to heal her emotions (instead of drawing the healing of the suffering area of her body), which meant being admitted into the group instead of being rejected and pushed *to the ground*. This was quite a valuable avenue to work on healing the issue involved here.

### Fourth drawing, quadrant #3: The transition (see Figure 11.16)

In this transition drawing, my client began by *lifting* the wall that was crushing her. The turquoise blue she applied manually with great care and gentleness, especially around the little girl in drawing #2, illustrated the sky as well as water. The wall turned into a dam, for support. The naked figure seemed to have passed through the healing quadrant to send energy to the wounded girl in quadrant #2. He seemed to be coming to help her. My client felt like she was in contact with the ground and *in the flow*. I believe that the therapeutic effect of this drawing lies in my client's gesture to take care, to look after and to surround the wounded person with much gentleness. However, it was the whole previous process (awareness of feeling, catharsis, and liberation of the body) that gave her strength and allowed for the self-care action at that point.

After the four-quadrants exercise, my client made a connection: over the past few days, her left leg was weaker, and there was a lot of unexpressed fear of being disabled again by her disk herniation. The impression that she was falling into the same vicious circle was very strong.

I believe that through the four-quadrants process she had access to a part of herself unable to self-express until now: the young wounded girl with a deep feeling of exclusion, incomprehension and even injustice. Now, she could progress towards healing that part of herself which was unable

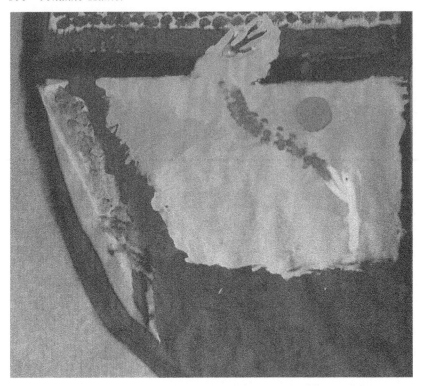

*Figure 11.16* (Fourth drawing, quadrant #3) *The transition.* About 15 inches x 15
inches (about 38 cm x 38 cm). Tempera.

to speak, and this part could truly be reconnected with her consciousness
and body.

Here is what this client said about how that exercise impacted her pains,
one year after the session:

> 'The exercise had the effect of eliminating the painful dorsal point in
> my back and it never returned. It decreased right after drawing and
> speaking and then disappeared completely in the next few days. I
> know I did not do any specific physical exercises for this during this
> time. I personally think that this decrease only resulted from the four-
> quadrants exercise. In terms of hernia pains, they also lessened, and
> my leg gained strength. It seems to me that repeating the exercise
> would be beneficial. At another time, I also drew a twisting sensation
> in my back, which was reflected in my posture. After quadrant #4, it
> decreased a lot then disappeared completely in the next days, and it
> also never returned'.

Figure 11.17 shows all of the four quadrants:

***Quadrant # 2 Quadrant # 1***

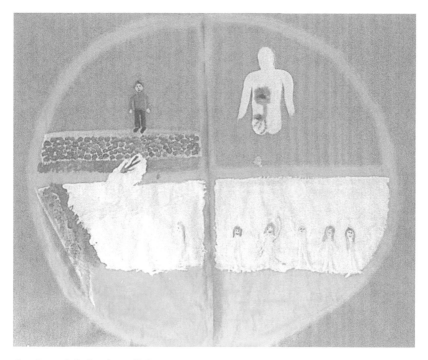

***Quadrant # 3 Quadrant # 4***
*Figure 11.17* The four-quadrants mandala. 5 feet x 5 feet (1.52 m x 1.52 m).
Tempera.

## Case study E

### *Chronic cervicalgia*

This client, a 51-year-old art therapy student, works on a chronic neck
pain that has been going on for over 15 years and was relatively under
control. Her whole process during the six-day intensive week is presented here, showing what she took away from the four-quadrants exercise, while framing this work within her whole journey and her issues.
This story highlights the importance of the work involved through this

exercise, while also considering the whole workshop's results. It also helps the viewer to grasp the importance of the 'temenos', a therapeutic setting where the participants feel safe enough for such a deep self-exploration. Safety is essentially the responsibility of the art therapist.

Here is what this student wrote about her process:

> The week before the workshop, I had a sudden and significant neck pain, the untypical length and intensity of which forced me to take medication and seek chiropractic care. This "coincidence" would feed my work and serve as a reference during the workshop.
>
> For the first experiential process, we were asked to give shape to the body sensations using forms, lines and colours within a fullsize body. I

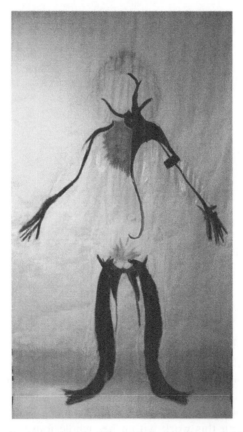

*Figure 11.18* The fragmented body. 5 feet x 8 feet (1.52 m x 2.44 m). Mix media.

got in touch with painful areas of contraction and tension, as well as frustration, fatigue and an urgent need to rest (to relax). Serving as 'X-rays' showing healthy areas and unwell areas, my drawings confirmed that the key problem areas were the nape and the left shoulder, within the structure formed by the spine and muscles, particularly the trapezius muscle. I called this drawing 'The fragmented body' (see Figure 11.18).

On the second day, we were invited to make a giant mandala divided into four quadrants (see Figure 11.19).

### First drawing, quadrant #1: The painful sensation

For the first quadrant, I decided to go deeper into what is going on with my upper back. I drew the sensation felt in this area in superimposed layers and overlapping forms, which abruptly brought back memories of my mother's demands in my youth.

### Second drawing, quadrant #2: The past origin of the pain

The second quadrant, which was about drawing the first time this sensation was felt, allowed me to explore these feelings more deeply. As my discomfort had no connection with any specific trauma or disease, my guess was that my pain dated back to my first torticollis, around the age of ten. I drew myself as a well-bred girl in a setting that spontaneously took shape: a house becoming a school, then a church. It was all in there: the demands of parental education, school, and religion.

### Third drawing, quadrant #4: The healing

In the fourth quadrant, I drew the sense of well-being that the healing or the relaxation of tensions would bring – light open spaces having the color of the light rays in a rainbow.[2]

### Fourth drawing, quadrant #3: The transition

The third quadrant bridged the gap between this well-being and the tensions, indicating a progressive healing, as well as lighter colours and elongated forms.

**Quadrant #2   Quadrant #1**

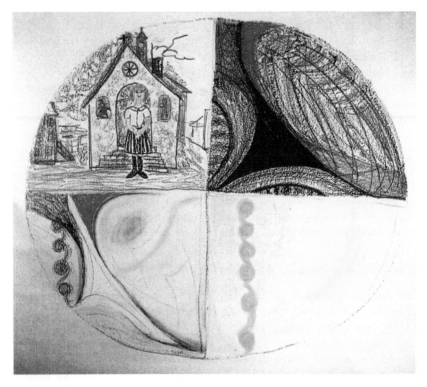

**Quadrant # 3   Quadrant # 4**
Figure 11.19 The four-quadrants mandala. 5 feet x 5 feet (1.52 m x 1.52 m). Mix media.

The following night, I had a dream where I saw how violent I was against myself, and that I did not allow myself to take up space. This dream and the drawing of the previous day helped me to understand that symbolically, the left side of my body, which was often painful, was bullied by my rational side which imposed its rhythm and will upon it. This realization paved the way for the next experiential process. This time, the artwork consisted of a large scribble based on the inner sensation and movement. I first experienced a feeling of annoyance and tingling in my limbs. Lines were first zigzagged then traced in a teeter-totter movement and in expanding large circular lines, which I enjoyed a lot. Traced using both hands, these large semicircular lines were then transferred onto the next sheet and completed with a few lines drawn in scroll forms, as my energy was slowly harmonizing.

When I looked at the scribble, I saw a little girl who seemed like a difficult child, with her hair a mess and a crooked mouth. I was both surprised and bothered by the caricatured style, wondering if I was still engaged in the art therapy process or just trivializing. During the small group sharing that followed, I realized that it was part of the art therapy process, because the little girl with a sharp mind, great vitality, independence, and leadership who had just come out of the closet was the complete opposite of the wise and submissive girl drawn the day before. She needed to take up space (interestingly...), to make friends and, more than anything, to allow herself not to be perfect. I am pleased to call this figure dis-introjected, and she shall be christened 'Pippa Longstocking, the Bad Girl on the block', commonly known as 'The Little Pest' (see Figure 11.20).

This new character had demands and raised fears; the following night, I dreamt that my father was dying and I was missing the lullabies of my mother who passed away earlier. In reality, my parents are still alive and in their eighties, so the dream was about the fear of my inner little girl to lose her parents' support if she would let herself be a *little pest!* In the next

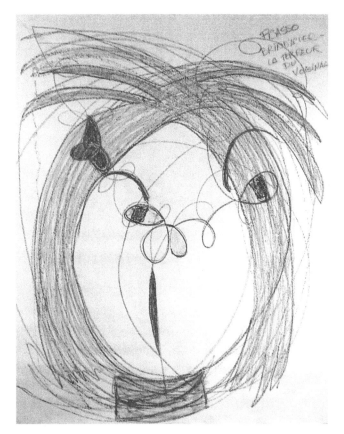

*Figure 11.20* Pippa Longstocking, the Bad Girl on the block or Little Pest. 5 feet x 5 feet (1.52 m x 1.52 m). Drawing pencils and oil pastels.

two days, I also went through moments when I strongly felt the fear of losing my friends if I was exuberant and took up too much space.

I approached the fourth experiential process in this state of mind. I was instructed to draw another area of the body where I felt discomfort or pain and to do *hands-on healing* on it (see Figure 11.21). This time, I worked on the tension in my upper back combined with chest congestion and a knot in the upper sternum. On a second sheet, I enlarged the sensation and it took shape in dark colors: black, blue, purple, and dark green. While I was drawing, I realized that my left arm was hot and hurting. Then, I applied gouache of a clear aqua colour on the whole surface of the sheet. It felt like covering the pain with clay plaster. I was using a big brush for broad brushstrokes. A few minutes later, I noticed with astonishment and pleasure that I was breathing more comfortably. The painful knot, however, had not gone away – in my mind, pink felt like the best choice after considering various colours. So I covered this area with pink tissue paper, giving it a heart-shaped texture and adding a small

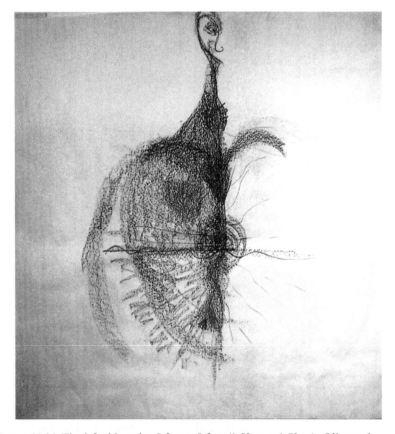

*Figure 11.21* The left side pain. 5 feet x 5 feet (1.52 m x 1.52 m). Oil pastels.

yellow mass in the center as a symbol for light. The knot untied. I was touched when I heard my inner voice saying that this area was not sick, it just needed to be taken into consideration given its importance to me. A little later, I realized that this area was home to the heart chakra. The next night, my dream reflected the healing theme and illustrated that 'things can be rather simple and work', as an offset for the *perfect little girl* valuing complicated schemes.

In conclusion, in order for the child that I had been to meet all educational, societal, and religious expectations, my back, my neck, and my shoulders turned stiff. In fact, I was just trying to do *the right thing* in order to be valued and loved, but by doing so I lost touch with my soul and gradually shed my true nature and my vitality. The body remained imprinted with these tensions and now had a chance to break free.

Although the pain returned occasionally one year after the workshop owing to a poor alignment of my cervical vertebrae, I learned that allowing the 'Little Pest' to take up more space was beneficial for my well-being. For example, I woke up with neck pain symptoms on a June morning. In the following hours, I had the chance to take a strong stand and speak up to a police officer who prevented me from going back home, because of a priority activity on public roads. When I arrived home, I was angry and not particularly proud of my actions, but my neck was less painful...

## Notes

1 This case study was first published in 2001 in *Revue Québécoise de Psychologie*, Vol. *22(1)*, 33–48.
2 Author's note: As my years of experience accumulated, I began to always ask clients and students to draw the healing in the same body parts as drawn in the first quadrant, to ensure a more specific healing experience. For the client in case study E, the information provided is still meaningful, indicating a need to break free from too constricting cultural norms. However, in many other cases, the information was not significant enough if they simply drew a positive feeling in the fourth quadrant.

# 12 Somatic Art Therapy and Chronic Pain
## Case Studies

*Johanne Hamel*

Three examples are presented in this chapter: two are psychotherapies of one and three years respectively (examples A and C), and the other one is a unique session for an acute whiplash symptom (example B). The first two (A and B) focus on pain associated with procedural memories as a result of motor vehicle accidents. Case study (C) is about chronic pain successfully treated with somatic art therapy, in a context of multiple stresses.

### Case study A: Back pain following a motor vehicle accident − access to procedural memory

My 48-year-old client had a severe motor vehicle accident four months earlier. The physicians concluded that she suffered from chronic pain, as nothing could explain the pain from a medical perspective. I saw her in art therapy sessions once a week for a year during the first eight months, then every two weeks to facilitate her return to work, for a total of 40 sessions of one hour each. Initially, my clinical observations were as follows.

There was a deep sense of loss of integrity owing to:

- A questioning of her identity following the accident trauma
- A feeling of psychological discomfort caused by the identity de-structuration
- A questioning of her fundamental values, for example the role of work in her life
- Having to cope with physical losses or with temporary or chronic mental incapacities, such as difficulty concentrating, lower energy levels, decreasing autonomy and chronic pain
- Having to readjust to a new physical and psychological reality brought a feeling of being on the verge of a new life cycle

Moreover, additional issues and needs emerged during the evaluation period:

- To better articulate her own needs and become more assertive on an emotional level, among other things
- To be less demanding of herself

- To break away from her parents' life experience on a psychological level in order to make her own choices, especially in terms of their experience as a couple.

All the topics mentioned above were worked on in the one-year process. Three sessions focusing specifically on chronic pain were conducted five months after the accident. Although the six-month criterion for diagnosing chronic pain was not met, there was nothing that might medically explain or ease the pain from her physicians' perspective.

The three sessions on her chronic pain have successfully brought almost complete relief from pain. Using somatic art therapy, I was able to observe, just like Scaer (2001), that the pain was either related to the *procedural memory* or the *somatic memory* of the shock during the accident and, more specifically, to the attempt by the body to protect itself. During the sessions, the client understood that her body kept experiencing the accident, ignoring that it was over, as if time had frozen still. Through art therapy, we found a way to communicate with the body so that it could find relief. The discussion below explains how we made it in three sessions only.

### Session #1: The pain: the art process therapy approach

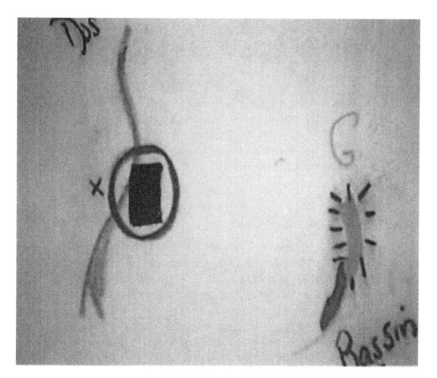

*Figure 12.1* (First drawing, first session) *The pain.* 18 inches x 24 inches (45 cm x 60 cm). Dry pastels.

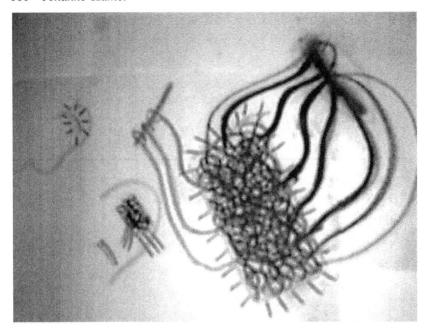

*Figure 12.2* (Second drawing, first session) *The pain amplified.* 18 inches x 24 inches (45 cm x 60 cm). Dry pastels.

The client was working on chronic pains at the iliac crest (groin pain). The first drawing (see Figure 12.1) shows where the pain was felt in the pelvis.

In the second drawing of the same session (see Figure 12.2), she enlarged the painful point (rectangle) and looked *into it*. She saw that it was filled with knots, that muscles were entangled and in disarray, still trying to protect the pelvic bones. Then she drew the point where muscles were supposed to be attached (lines on the left and right sides of the rectangle) and she tidied this up. In the third drawing (not illustrated), there were no more knots.

### Session #2: The pain: the silhouette

For this session, the client was still working on her chronic pain in the lower back. She first developed a sketch representing the point in her body where tension was felt (see Figure 12.3), then she enlarged the painful area. She realized that the muscles were trying to protect her endangered body, by contracting to lessen the vulnerable area: pressure was being exerted on that area (Figure 12.4, right drawing: arrows over and under the square, pushing in opposite directions). Then she drew the area gradually relaxing (see Figure 12.4: middle drawing: pale yellow arrows making space, and then she affirmed that muscles should be working in

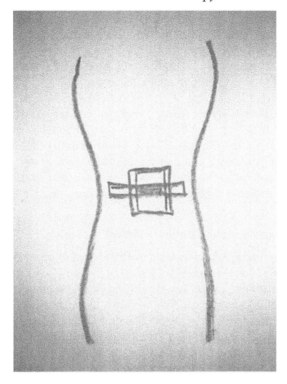

*Figure 12.3* (First drawing, second session) *The location of pain.* 18 inches x 24 inches (45 cm x 60 cm). Dry pastels.

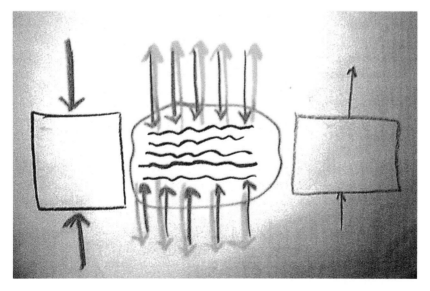

*Figure 12.4* (Second drawing, second session) *The pain amplified and pressure exerted.* 18 inches x 24 inches (45 cm x 60 cm). Dry pastels.

the same direction (see Figure 12.4: arrows around the left square). Finally, using the hands-on healing technique, she applied a soothing blue-green colour on the tense area (not shown here).

After the second session, the client reported a 90% decrease in pain, which never returned to its previous intensity.

In the following week, during a psychotherapy session, she was able to articulate quite intensively her fear of dying or becoming paralyzed as a result of the accident. It was the first time that she got in touch with these fears with such clarity. I think that this occurred in the aftermath of the somatic work done in the previous week and that it might have contributed to the almost complete suppression of the chronic pain. Indeed, she noticed a decrease in restlessness, which she had been feeling ever since the accident.

### Session #3: The pain: the art process therapy approach

Physical pain is generally associated with unarticulated intense emotions, which prevent physical relaxation. This next somatic work on the client's spine, one year almost to the day after the accident, seemed to confirm this idea. At that time, she wanted to work on a cracking sound that she was sometimes hearing in her lower back. She drew the vertebrae of her column and the cracking sensation like a small explosion in her back (not shown here). She felt that one vertebra was cracked and became aware of very strong feelings related to the event: the fear of being dislocated by the impact at the time of the accident, as well as the fear of what could have happened to her. She explicitly made a drawing of the vertebra in her spine and the firm nerve inside (session drawings not shown here). She immediately had feelings of gentleness and well-being. She applied a healing color all over the drawing (not shown here). Following that work, she never heard the cracking sound again. The soothing effect is likely to have resulted from this unconscious emotion having been brought to light and expressed.

My client's work during these few sessions confirm Scaer's (2001) theories on procedural memory.

## Case study B: A brief example of whiplash symptoms

Following a motor vehicle accident, a 47-year-old client was experiencing shoulder pain, difficulty in concentrating and headaches. In the therapy session two days after the event, she illustrated the pain (See Figure 12.5) then amplified the knot at the core of her pain (see Figure 12.6) so as to explore and amplify its content.

As there were alternating upward and downward lines within the knot, the lines pointing upwards then those pointing downwards were explored one after the other, then reproduced repeatedly until the patient could understand what these lines meant (see Figure 12.7).

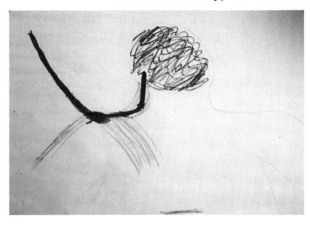

*Figure 12.5  The shoulder pain.* 18 inches x 24 inches (45 cm x 60 cm). Oil pastels.

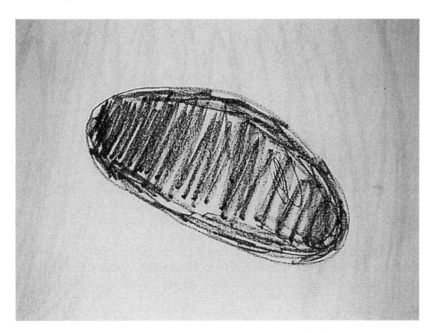

*Figure 12.6  The knot at the core of the pain.* 18 inches x 24 inches (45 cm x 60 cm). Oil pastels.

The upward lines lead the client to become aware of feelings of anger regarding a friend, among others, who showed greater concern about the damage to the car than about her injuries at the time of the accident. Exploring the downward lines revealed her tendency to be gentle, to repress anger, and not to speak her mind. For the last drawing (not illustrated here),

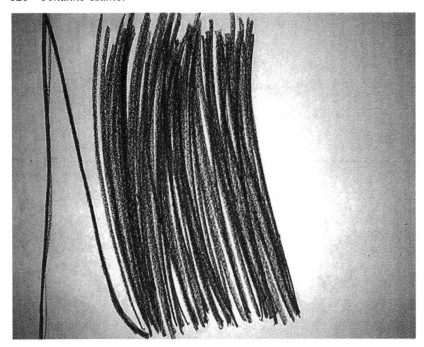

*Figure 12.7 Lines within the pain knot.* 18 inches x 24 inches (45 cm x 60 cm). Oil
    pastels.

she used the hands-on healing approach. Using gouache, she applied a blue
colour on the first drawing, which produced inner calm, reduced restlessness,
and soothed the pain right away. The next day, the client had a cortisone
treatment that completely eliminated the pain, making it impossible to assess
the impact of our art therapy work in the longer term. However, it is interesting to note that the patient experienced effects in the shoulder during the
session itself. Headaches and difficulty concentrating might be worked on in
art therapy as well. As a result of this session, my client was able to express
her anger to the individuals concerned and develop more and more self-
assertiveness, which also helped to reduce her headaches.

### Case story C: Acquired dyspareunia, a process art psychotherapy treatment

This case is about a 31-year-old client who attended art psychotherapy sessions with me for three years. He presented with symptoms of generalized
acquired dyspareunia (painful testicles) as a result of psychological factors.
Clinical examinations revealed no medical condition, and no substance was
involved in the etiology of the pain.

On his first visit, he had been suffering from pain in testicles for two years;
he had tried a large number of alternative treatments including acupuncture,

chiropractic care, homeopathy, osteopathy, essential oils, Filipino healing, and a more traditional talk psychotherapy based on an eclectic approach. Nobody could explain or stop the pain, which he sometimes described as excruciating, occurring at any time, sometimes in connection with sex, but not always. Of course, he had undergone all the necessary medical tests, and nothing had been discovered. When I saw him for the first time, the pain was so intense that he was walking with difficulty.

The other reasons for consulting a psychotherapist included a lot of stressors over the last two or three years: his father's death two years ago, burnout in the last three years, followed by a career change, health problems of one of his children, separation from his wife nine months earlier, and a new romantic relationship for the past two months. There was also great tension in the relationship with his mother.

One year after the beginning of the art therapy process, including a three-month break during the summer, symptoms cleared up and did not return. We explored the pain from all angles. We worked regularly on his night dreams and often used, during the first months, the art therapy process approach where one draws the sensation of pain, representing it by lines, forms, and colors. We ended up discovering that his pain came from a set of subjective factors and physical processes that I would summarize with the following images, which were gradually revealed through his successive drawings, art creations, and dreams:

- First, because of a set of circumstances related to his financial situation and paternal inheritance, the idea that his mother basically *got him by the balls* since the death of his father, given that he was financially dependent on her. This situation ended one year after the start of the therapy, when he talked to his mother about this, as discussed in therapy; it matched the time that the pain cleared up
- An image of sexual guilt from an extramarital affair he had before separating
- The fear of procreating with his new partner, whereas his two-year-old child had been very sick, which he had painfully experienced physically
- And most of all, a vision of masculinity where emotions are repressed and where emotional life relates only to sexuality. Every painful emotion was felt in the genital system, creating pain. Both the resentment towards his mother and the guilt or fear of procreating presented themselves this way. As the therapy process went along, we noticed that the site of psychic and physical pain was shifting. After withdrawing from the testicles, the pain presented itself as discomfort felt in the chest, and then higher and higher up to the throat. It was almost as though the emotions, increasingly getting through to the conscious mind, were being felt higher and higher up in the body, giving rise to images more and more easily interpreted

This is how my client got in touch with his great fear of being abandoned and was able to see his emotional dependency on his new partner. As he became aware of his emotions and emotional needs and expressed them much more quickly, these processes stopped manifesting as painful physical symptoms. He ended up feeling as if his body was talking to him, as long as he was willing to listen. Indeed, he developed a greater receptivity to his proprioceptive processes; he said that he would know right away whether a situation generated emotional tension for him, by staying attentive to his inner sensations.

In one year of art therapy, the chronic pain cleared up. Two factors participated in his healing: the treatment of the psychological suffering underlying the physical pain and the familiarization with interoceptive sensations.

# 13  A Healing Metaphor

*Patcharin Sughondhabirom*

Johanne Hamel is my respected teacher. Since 2017, when she came to teach art therapy to students in Thailand in a collaborative project between CiiAT[1] and IPATT[2], in which I am the local director, I discovered a new horizon of the art therapy field. Johanne has shown me somatic art therapy tools and techniques that brought art therapy to another level of practice. I have learnt so much since then. When Johanne invited me to share in this book my intervention with a student while participating in her six-day intensive workshop 'Somatic art therapy', I felt more than honored.

As an assistant, I observed that participants in her workshop had a good opportunity to witness the transformative power of somatic art therapy in their own process. Most were able to give meanings to their own pain and suffering and were eventually able to transform themselves into a healthier person with less somatic pain.

This chapter will be a case presentation of a somatic art therapy work, observing every possible aspects of a metaphoric intervention on chronic pains, including the retrieving of implicit memories to which we do not usually have conscious access. We will make this case study anonymous by using the pseudo name *Joy* when referring to this participant. We intend to protect the person by keeping personal information highly confidential and by asking every participant in the group to do the same. We are grateful that Joy gave us permission to reveal her images and personal story.

Joy has been suffering from chronic pain since her childhood. She is now a medical doctor pursuing art therapy training. In her mid-forties, Joy has a slim body with long limbs. With the look of a teenager in a T-shirt and jeans, she appears to be keen and nimble.

## First day of the workshop: The life-size silhouette

On the very first day of the somatic art therapy workshop, Johanne asked participants to draw their somatic sensations in a full-size body silhouette. This assignment insists on the importance of representing inner sensations as they are subjectively felt from within, which is the very definition of *soma* (Hamel, 2014). Joy painted her whole body with heavy red and black colours illustrating her somatic chronic pain in her right arm, her back, her right bottom, right leg, and right foot (see Figure 13.1).

We were shocked how contrasted it was from her external appearance. She told us that these sensations were chronic and had affected almost her

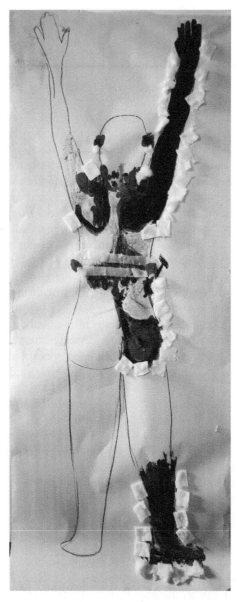

*Figure 13.1 The silhouette.* 34 inches x 80 inches (85 cm x 195 cm). Mixed media, tempera on 50 pounds (80 g/m) paper, cotton pads and, sewing threads.

whole body. She had gone through many investigations and received all kinds of medical treatments, including modern techniques such as oral medicine, skin graft surgery for her leg, cervical traction and ultrasound therapy for her shoulders, and alternative medicine such as acupuncture. After all that, the intensity of the pain reduced only a little.

Taking a closer look, I saw in her artwork sharp objects pricking and making holes inside the foot of her silhouette and many stitches tied to the tearing wounds on the foot and the calf (see Figure 13.2). It was painful for me to see so many symbolic damages on her body.

This reminded me of similar situations that I had witnessed when I was working as a medical doctor many years ago. It gave me a sense of emergency. The participant must have felt it too, as she responded to her own feelings by putting cotton pads as a cushion, an attempt to comfort the foot, which was at least what she could do at that time to relieve her pain. Such a symbolic act on the soma could result many times in a real relief in the body part.

As Joy has a degree in medicine, we believe that her own medical knowledge prompted her to do some stitching to the wounds, as we can see it better here on the painted calf (see Figure 13.3). The sense of emergency was rushing to both of us, as we share similar background in medical fields. When a patient comes with multiple injuries and massive bleeding similar to what is illustrated here, our responses are automatic, immediate, and full.

As an observer, I was impressed that Joy had so much courage to attend to all these pains in her body. Being a student in art therapy, she knew that physical pains are connected with emotional pains. Relieving an emotional pain connected to a physical one will reduce the pain sensation of up to 70–80% if the client is willing to face the emotional component and

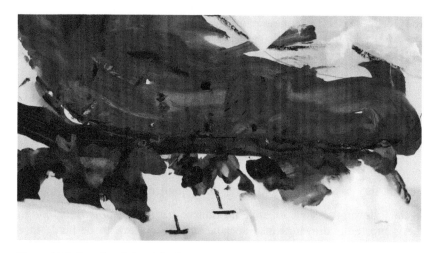

*Figure 13.2* Details of the right foot

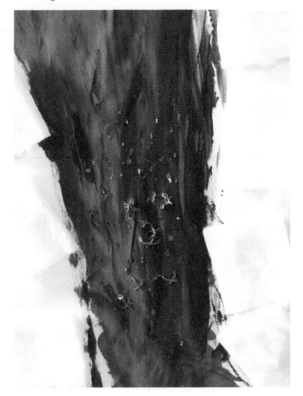

*Figure 13.3* Details of the calf

express it fully (Church, 2013). This revisiting was not easy, but she was willing to face her pains with a hope of understanding and healing them and freeing herself from these pains that bothered her for almost all of her life. After the full-size body silhouette was done, Joy shared with the group with tears in her eyes that these sensations had been with her since she was very young.

During those six days in the workshop, she appeared to be highly alert, super sensitive, and seemed to have a higher ability to access some pre-verbal or traumatic memories. We know from neurosciences that these kinds of memory are not readily available, being mostly stored in the implicit memories of the right brain structures (Hamel, 2016).

## Second day of the workshop: The 'four-quadrants' method

In the following session, Johanne introduced her *four-quadrants method* to the group. Four drawings in a specific succession have to be made in a specific way, inside a giant circle. As a reminder, in chapter 10, she describes her method in this way:

*First drawing*: The instruction is to draw a current or often present physical pain, focusing specifically on the painful *sensation*.

*Second drawing*: The instruction is to go back in time until a similar sensation was felt for the very first time.

*Third drawing*: The participant is asked to draw how it would feel if this part of the body was completely healed and healthy.

*Fourth drawing*: For the last drawing, the instruction is to represent the transition between the first drawing (pain) and the third one (healing), usually by borrowing visual features from the images drawn in both or by expressing emotions repressed during the events portrayed in the second drawing.

In her own words, Hamel says: 'The effect of this four-step approach is to grasp the existential message of a pain (quadrant 1), to understand where the pain originates from (quadrant 2), to acknowledge what is possible (quadrant 4) and to understand how healing can be achieved (quadrant 3)' (See chapter 10).

In my own understanding, the *four-quadrants method* that Hamel developed is a very good example of a practical interpretation of the Four Noble Truths of Buddhism[3] (Gold and Zahm, 2018). It is incredible to see the correlation between each quadrant in Hamel's method and each of the Noble Truths in Buddha's teaching. My way of viewing this is more like a comparative religion study. The first quadrant of Hamel's, where one needs to admit that one is suffering and one needs to describe through the arts what the suffering looks like and where it is situated in the body, is related to the first Noble Truth: Dukkha, which is when a Buddhist is asked to define her/his own suffering. The second quadrant, where one needs to go back in time, to find an event in which the sensation appeared for the first time and to portray it onto the paper is related to the second Noble Truth: Samudaya, which is when a Buddhist searches for meaning of her/his own suffering. The possibility to understand the origin of the suffering lies in there, in the art forms through Hamel's method and in conceptual thinking forms through the practice of Buddhism. The fourth quadrant, where one is asked to imagine what the body part will look like when the suffering is gone is related to the third Noble Truth: Nirodha, which is the state of mind when a Buddhist is free from suffering. And the third quadrant, where one searches inside oneself what needs to be done to achieve the healing portrayed in the fourth quadrant is related to the fourth Noble Truth: Magga, which are the Buddhist paths of transformation. It feels as if Hamel literally translated each of the Noble Truths into art therapy process, even though she had not heard of the Four Noble Truths of Buddhism before. Her four-quadrant intervention is original and effective. This surprising correlation made me wonder if her connectedness with Buddha and his teaching had begun a lot earlier than we could plausibly imagine.

## First drawing, quadrant #1: The painful sensation

That day, for the first quadrant, Joy chose to work on the sensation on her right shoulder in which she felt a burning and piercing sensation, as shown on the right upper piece of the mandala (See Figure 13.4, first drawing, quadrant #1).

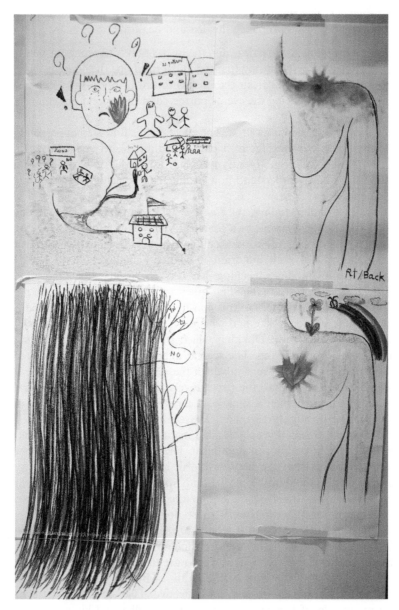

*Figure 13.4* The four quadrants, 44 inches x 58 inches (110 cm x 145 cm). Oil pastels on 100 pounds (160 g/m) drawing paper.

### Second drawing, quadrant #2: The past origin of the pain

At first Joy could not understand the meaning of the sensation, but when Johanne guided the students through relaxation and meditation to go back to the very first time that they felt this sensation, she found a piece of memory in school when she was bullied and slapped on the face (see Figure 13.4, second drawing, quadrant #2 on the left upper section). In somatic art therapy, we believe that the first event is usually the origin of the emotional pain lodged in a body part.

Moreover, Joy remembered she went to her loving father and was surprisingly disappointed by his response. At that time, what happened to her was not taken seriously. Instead of taking action against the bully, her parents minimized it. Joy believed that her father made a compromise to make things easier for the headmaster, to avoid any future trouble. She felt that her emotional pain was completely ignored.

### Third drawing, quadrant #4: The healing

In her third drawing (see Figure 13.4, quadrant #4 on the right lower section), she imagined what it would feel like if the shoulder was healed. She turned the dark painful burning spot on her shoulder into a seed of love budding and blooming and added a rainbow on its side.

### Fourth drawing, quadrant #3: The transition

When working on her fourth drawing, the transition from pain to healing, in order to get the body part healed eventually, she felt that she needed to express her anger for the healing to occur (See Figure 13.4, quadrant #3 on the left lower section: the black lines). As Hamel once said, repressed emotions, especially anger, lodged somewhere in the body and causing unexplainable sensations, are difficult to acknowledge. In addition, for many cultures in Asia, including Thailand, these emotions are often perceived as unacceptable. The fact that Joy was able to sense this specific need and respond to it without censoring was a triumph. This is an evidence of the intuition winning over the intellect. As a therapist, it was a pleasure to see this process.

Underneath the anger lines, there were hands with the word 'NO' on each finger in both Thai and in English. Those were Joy's hands desperately trying to stop all the abuses: physical and emotional abuse by her classmates; and emotional and power abuse by the adults. The anger lines were directed specifically towards the school headmaster who took the events as no more than children playing and said that it was not a big deal. Joy thought that the headmaster was unjust because he took the side of the abuser who was the daughter of his close friend.

At this point, Johanne gave a suggestion to Joy to remove the dark spot, even though it was transformed into a seed of love because, visually, this shape was still sharp and pointing into the body, symbolically hurting the shoulder. It was not safe to leave such thing in the body, as it is actually a retroflection of one's anger on the self (Gold and Zahm, 2018). We knew that more work needed to be done to heal the pain.

### Third day of the workshop: A giant scribble

In the next session, a giant scribble exercise is introduced in the workshop to allow some inner wisdom to come up from the unconscious. Joy created the shape of an hourglass from her giant scribble (see Figure 13.5 A). The hourglass looked like it was about to fall. When allowed to manipulate the piece, Joy turned the paper upside down to stabilize it. Then she added some colour to it and its surroundings (see Figure 13.5 B). The ground was created with a solid dark purple.

Outside the hourglass were petals of red flower supporting the inside. She also created a pointy apparatus on the side of the hourglass, a weapon to protect herself (see Figure 13.5 B). Again, I was impressed by her intuition and her spontaneity in responding to her own feelings. I believe that part of it resulted from the previous process when she learned that in time of crisis, nobody else was really there for her. She had been completely on her own dealing with the abuses. As an adult looking back into that memory, Joy might have wondered what she could do to protect herself.

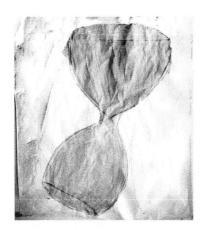 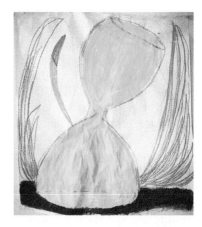

*Figure 13.5A The hourglass shape.* 34 inches x 34 inches (75 cm x 75 cm). Pencil on 50 pounds (80 g/m) paper.

*Figure 13.5B The stable hourglass shape.* 34 inches x 34 inches (75 cm x 75 cm). Mixed media including acrylic paints and oil pastels.

That day, I saw in her creation that Joy was becoming self-reliant. In the art making, she demonstrated that she was able to sense the insecurity in her environment. She understood her needs to establish stability and responded to her needs by turning the hourglass upside down and giving a solid ground for the piece to sit on. She developed strategies to care for herself by adding layers of petal around the hourglass and creating a weapon to protect it. I felt delighted that Joy was advancing in a positive and constructive direction. It was important because the possibility for her to heal was thus growing in my therapist's mind. Becoming intuitive and more self-reliant, Joy was developing the kinds of strengths that she needed for the next challenges. Without any clues on the intensity of what was to follow, she was already on the path to heal herself and was well equipped.

## Fourth day of the workshop: Exploring a burning sensation

After day three of the workshop, I noticed some changes in Joy's behavior. She seemed to be flooded by many childhood memories. A burning sensation on her face was growing and expanding to both sides. In the next session, Joy chose to work with the burning sensation on both cheeks (see Figure 13.6). She explored the sensation through different shades of red, orange, and yellow. Then another piece of memory came. When Joy was a child, her mother hired a nanny to look after her. One day when Joy was

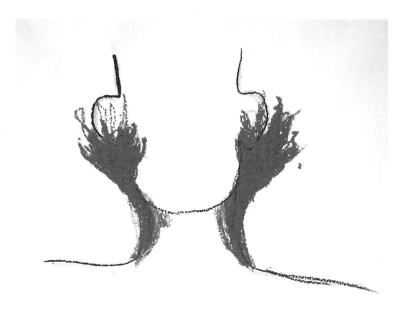

*Figure 13.6 The burning sensation.* 24 inches x 29 inches (60 cm x 82½ cm). Oil pastels on 100 pounds (160 g/m) drawing paper.

about one year old, she was left unattended. She accidentally hit a boiling pot, and the boiling water was spilled over onto her right leg.

The burnt wound was severe and caused a huge scar even after receiving all available treatments, including a skin graft that her mother actively requested. I was able to see the relation between the present sensation in her cheeks and the sensation on her right leg derived from the accident in the far past. It was astonishing to see the burning sensation traveling from the leg to the cheeks and bringing this traumatic memory to the conscious level and to her immediate attention. In the past, the adults in her family told Joy repeatedly that the scar was her own fault, even though it was actually caused by the neglectful behavior of the nanny. Joy was ashamed of her scarred legs and tended to hide them from people's eyes.

However, the nanny stayed in the family ever since and still is. Joy could not understand why she did not like her nanny until this piece of memory came back to her in the workshop. The mother often told Joy to let go of her negative feelings towards the nanny, for her own sake, in order to have peace of mind. However, Joy understood that the mother had said that to keep the working nanny, for her own convenience. This idea brought to Joy another feeling, a sense of betrayal. The mother was someone she completely trusted, someone who was supposed to protect her from danger and harm. However, she was the one who decided to keep the neglectful nanny, which meant that Joy had unnecessarily been put at risk again at a very young age. At that point, Joy was deeply sad, angry, and disappointed. Tears flooded into her eyes relentlessly. She felt engulfed in a loop of distress, and the feeling of disappointment was becoming more intense. She felt badly hurt.

She looked at her full-size body silhouette and felt hopeless. The emotional damage seemed to be massive and out of control. It was overwhelming to me as well. My heart was pumping fast, and my muscles were tense. I felt that I needed to help this person, to alleviate her intense pain. My intuition told me that it was time to take care of this frail person. I looked at the full-size body silhouette and again felt overwhelmed by the size of the injury. The body parts that were covered with dark heavy colour looked like dead tissue to me (dry gangrene, in medical terms).

If this happened in an emergency room, we would need to explore under the dead skin and find out if we could keep these body parts and the bones underneath. As the patient could still feel the pain in the arms and legs, I imagined that we would see pink living flesh and bones underneath, if we were in a real emergency room. Then we would need to do a deep cleaning to remove germs and debris out of the wound. In the end, we would apply some antibiotic gel and create a good environment for the new flesh to grow by itself. But in a real medical setting, the size of the wound of my patient would have worried me. It could take forever for the new flesh to grow back and to cover this huge skin lost. The words 'skin graft surgery' came to my mind immediately.

## Fifth day of the workshop: A healing metaphor

I took on this idea and consulted with Johanne. At this point I felt like creating a medical healing metaphor for Joy's full-size body silhouette. In my medical opinion, skin graft surgery in real life heals more quickly, which means that the length of time for recovery after the treatment is more tolerable for most patients. These were dead wounds, and they could not heal if we did not remove the dead skin. On the technical parts, Johanne was concerned that this body silhouette was made on 80 grams/meter paper. She agreed that this kind of paper might not be able to hold more art materials, especially healing colours made from heavy tempera or acrylic paints. She asked me in a respectful manner what options we could possibly have in terms of symbolically healing this body. The artist inside myself suggested we add some strength to the 'body' first. We could use a sturdy sheet of brown paper that we had in our studio to give extra support to the whole body. When the body would be strong enough to tolerate the 'operation', we could remove the dead skin and do a skin graft. We would be able to apply healing colours onto the new material afterwards and let the new skin flap bridge with the 'flesh' underneath.

As it was day five, and we both were concerned about the time frame and the closing of the group on the next day, it did not feel right to postpone this opportunity to heal this body. Johanne cleverly split the workshop group into two parts. Johanne and a student assistant took the big group, and the other part was solely for me to work with Joy. I was touched by the amount of trust Johanne had in me. She gave me this wonderful opportunity to proceed with my ideas without any doubt in my ability and with complete trust in my suggestion of the medical metaphorical way of healing. I was nervous, as I had not used somatic art therapy methods with any clients before. I usually played with imagination when doing therapeutic work with small children. But this felt more like a serious play with adult in therapy. I took the opportunity anyway, being comfortable with Johanne's help next door if need be. I asked Joy to come with me in a separate studio space and told the rest of the group that I would not be available to assist them in the afternoon. Everybody received the message and nodded quietly.

Upon beginning the therapeutic work with Joy, I had in mind some structures that I wanted to use as healing metaphors for her suffering body. My imagination was playing a big part in creating different settings, different roles, and improvising the conversations. I closed the door, and we imagined that it was a door to an emergency room. We had just finished carrying an injured body inside the emergency room. We used the floor as an emergency table to do first aid. I communicated with Joy as if she was a medical colleague in hospital and gave Joy the leading role. In that imaginary space, Joy was quite spontaneous. We spoke doctor's language with technical terms that only the two of us could understand. The goal was for the two of us to team up and stabilize this injured body to be ready for the operation. At that point, I realized that I was giving Joy really hard work because she was the actual patient full of pain, and she had to split herself in two; another part of her became the doctor who gave treatment to her own body. I believe that it was crucial therapeutically that Joy as the patient would be able to decide how to heal herself. At the same time, I myself felt more alert and ready to take over if anything happened.

On the emergency table, we removed cotton pads soaked with blood (red tempera paint on the body), and we removed the remaining sharp objects (in the stitching done the first day on the silhouette). The 'body' felt delicate and frail when we touched the paper. Joy was very careful with each of her moves and was taking care of the body very respectfully. Then I suggested to her that this body needed extra bone strength. I told Joy that we happened to have a newly invented bony plate technology to help us to add strength to a human body and that the method was quite simple.

I showed the big sturdy brown paper to Joy and asked her to insert the sheet under the body. I gave Joy a pencil to trace the whole body on this brown paper. I gave her scissors to remove unused brown paper outside the body tracing. I gave her bone glue (TOA Latex glue) to apply between the frail body and the bone sheet. Then I gave Joy another sheet of 80 grams/meter white paper to use as the bottom skin layer. Joy took the pencil and did the body tracing again.

She removed the unused part and glued the new white sheet as the bottom layer to the body. While Joy was doing these procedures, she sensed it with her hands that this body was getting stronger. The three-layered paper body was, at this point, not easy to break. It had its own strength and was able to hold its own weight at some level. Joy looked more relaxed when she touched the body. I told Joy that it was wonderful for me to feel the strength under the skin layers. Joy nodded and looked happy with the strength that she added to herself. I gave her a small moment to be with the body before telling her that a member of staff from the operating room had just called. The room was

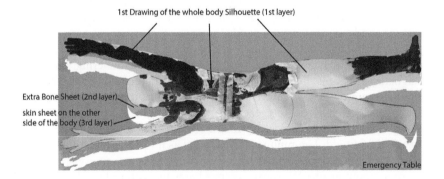

*Figure 13.7* The three layers of the body on the floor

ready for the skin graft operation. I asked if she was ready. Joy softly said yes with a gentle smile.

While she was sitting with the body on the floor, I put another sheet of white paper on a long table so that we could use it as an operating table. When Joy said yes, I told her to tell the body that we were about to bring her to an operating room for a surgical treatment, that there was nothing to be scared of, that the surgeons were highly skilled, that the bad skin would be removed so the healing could happen, and finally, that the anesthesia would be applied so that she would be asleep and would not feel any pain during the operation. Also, we would wake her up when everything was done, and afterwards she could still ask for a painkiller if she felt any pain or discomfort. Joy could not move her eyes away from the body. She looked as if she was in an altered state of mind!

When the table was ready, I made a gesture by inserting my two hands under the body's legs. Joy put her hands under the shoulders. I started counting 'one...two....three...' and up we lifted the three-layered paper body and transferred it onto the 'operating table'. Then I switched off all the lights except the one projecting its beam on the target table. It felt real to me, and I was completely ready to be a surgeon.

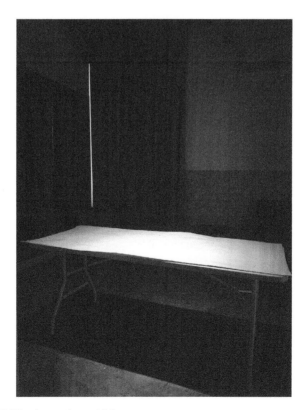

*Figure 13.8* The 'operating table'

But then, I changed my mind, remembering that therapeutically, it was better for Joy to be the surgeon, and so I stepped down and acted as her first assistant. While typing this chapter, I discovered that I had a desire to maximize therapeutic effect all along during this play, and making Joy 'the surgeon' means that she was in the best position to help herself. I guess I wanted to facilitate her implication in the process, even if at the time this decision was not that conscious.

In the operating room, I started a new conversation as if we had just come in and met each other for this operation. I called Joy 'Doctor' and introduced to her the idea that I would be her first assistant. I saw some shyness in her smile. I said to her that there was a lot of dead skin. It would probably take many hours to remove it. And it would take a lot longer for the skin to grow back and cover the lost surface. I asked her: 'What would you like to do? We could also do a skin grafting (I whispered).... Someone told me that an artificial skin flap from an international company has just arrived to our hospital this morning. It is the best one we have in the country. Would you like to use it for this patient?' A spark in Joy's eyes made me believe that she was completely in with me. Without hesitation, she responded in a clear and full sentence: *Yes, let's do the skin grafting.*

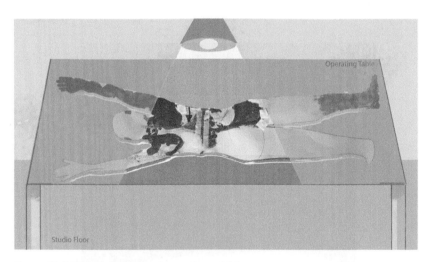

*Figure 13.9* The body on the 'operating table'

I grabbed the scissors and some clay sculpting tools from the shelf. Joy took the scissors in her right hand and another tool to use as a forceps in her left hand. She did not mind playing this role with me. She was pretty much at ease when cutting and removing the dead skin. When it was difficult to remove some piece, I handed her another sculpting tool that had a similar look to a surgical instrument (a curette) that surgeons use for scraping bad tissue. We continued to talk doctor's language in the operating field and renamed different art tools with surgical tool names.

When Joy inserted the blade (carving knife) underneath the arm, she discovered the bone sheet that she had added earlier. I saw a satisfaction and a sense of certainty in that moment. It would have given us a completely different experience if the bone sheet and the bottom sheet were not in there. She could have left a big hole, especially as it involved cutting the whole body part. Before the idea of skin grafting came, another possibility that came to mind was replacing this injured arm with an artificial arm piece. But that idea was too much to accommodate. In real life, if we did an amputation to remove the whole arm, we would be risking the patient with the other trauma of losing a body part. For that healing moment, I thought that Joy needed something gentle and kind. As I felt firmly connected with Joy, those feelings felt real to me, and I let those feelings guide me throughout the process.

When the dead skin on the arm was completely removed, I gave Joy another white sheet of paper that was long enough to cover the arm. 'Here it is, freshly baked, right out of the oven'. I presented this pretended skin flap to Joy with humor. She laughed a little before she took it from my hands. By that time, I felt the atmosphere had already become a little lighter. Joy appeared calm and relaxed. She was taking pleasure in caring for the body, being totally immersed in the experience. Time did not exist. Joy made sure that the skin flap was covering the wounded area. She used a pencil to trace the shape of the wound and then cut it with scissors. We placed the flap on the clean wound with some glue underneath.

We moved on to other parts that needed treatment and did similar procedures. When new flaps replaced all areas of dead skin, the whole body appeared mostly clean and really white. Joy started to apply the light green paint as a healing color on the part of the wound that did not need skin flap. I was on duty, serving the art materials that she wanted. As she asked for more green paint, and I realized that the bottle was almost empty, I asked her if she would accept similar remedy of the green healing medicine but from a different pharmaceutical company. Joy smiled openly and said yes. So I started mixing the paints, adding some white to tone down the intensity of the new green. The new color was not exactly the same green that she used before, but Joy was flexible enough to accept it.

With my eyes following the movement of her paintbrush, I stepped back and moved my focus on the whole body. I found myself wishing to see some skin color. This wish was unusually strong in my feeling, and I wondered if it had anything to do with my own psychic materials, or if it was simply an aesthetic concern for the body. Wanting the body to have some signs of aliveness within its skin, I told Joy that the patient looked really pale: 'She must have had a massive blood loss. Would you like to give her a blood transfusion?' Joy paused for a moment. She drew herself back a few steps to get a distant, holistic view of the person lying on the operating table. She looked at the whole body first and then looked at it again from head to toe. I guessed that she was probably having a conversation with herself. I then told myself that it should be ok if she did not want to add skin colour. I could explore this mysterious feeling later.

By the time that I finished a conversation with myself, Joy had finished hers too. She turned to me and said yes, she wanted to give this patient a blood transfusion. I said 'OK, I will ask the blood bank to send some in for her'. I was delighted inside and started to mix some paints to create skin color. I used a lot of white then added pink, orange, and a little bit of yellow for the color to be just like our Asian skin tone. Stirring the paints in a jar, I saw the skin color of a newly born baby, and I really liked it. Under the dim beam from that single light bulb, it was the colour of a baby only a few weeks old, when the skin is still translucent, and we see the baby's blood circulating underneath the skin. I presented that colour to Joy. With excitement, I told her that this was a skin colour of a new born and asked if she liked it, which she did. I admired her for being able to accept this and decided to keep that mysterious feeling to work on later for myself.

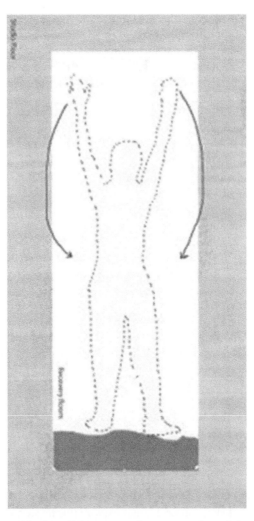

*Figure 13.10* Repositioning of the arms and reconstruction of the shoulders

Before Joy applied the paint, I asked if she wanted to reposition the two arms. She considered my suggestion briefly and then experimented with the arms. She tried bending them down. This new position added a relaxing feeling to the body. We reconstructed the shoulders to make them look proper with the hands down. Then Joy applied the skin colour on the white body parts. She seemed to enjoy the moment. Sometimes it felt as if she was patting the body repeatedly with a comforting gesture. She then decided to put new skin colour onto the whole body including the parts that had healing green colour on.

Now that the operation was done successfully, I started to form another plan inside my head. It took us altogether about an hour to do the resuscitation part in the emergency room and the skin graft surgery in the operating room. I looked at the clock and felt a need for at least 15 minutes more to complete the task. When Joy finished painting the skin, I asked her what kind of environment she wanted this person to wake up into. She had no specific idea, neither for the place nor for the environment. My suggestion for her was to close her eyes and think

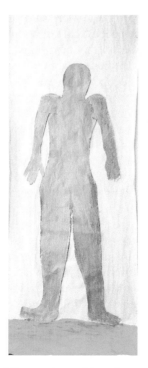

*Figure 13.11* Application of the new born skin colour and environment colours. 34 inches x 80 inches (85 cm x 195 cm). Mixed media including 50 pounds (80 g/m) white paper, 112 pounds (180 g/m) brown paper, acrylic paints, TOA Latex glue

about the kind of atmosphere that she wanted around this person. She found two words: love and lots of space. I asked what colours represented these two qualities for her. Joy said green and light blue. At this point, I already had a new white sheet prepared on the floor for the painting of the environment. I asked Joy to whisper to the body that the operation was done, and we were about to bring her to a recovery room. We would wake her up when she was ready. Again I counted 'one... two... three...', and up the body was lifted and transferred onto the new sheet on the floor, on which Joy could paint a nice environment for the body.

I went back to my collection of colours and offered her different shades of green. Joy told me that green represented love and she wanted 'leaf' green for the ground. She would like to cover the solid ground with soft grass for this person to stand on. For the blue, she wanted it very light like cool fresh air with some breeze and not too windy. Joy finished the whole painting in a reasonable time.

Joy stepped back to have the first look of the whole person in the new environment (see Figure 13.11). She took a quiet moment looking at this new body then turned to me with excitement in her eyes. Pointing to the raising shoulders (see Figure 13.11) she said 'This person is breathing, taking in the fresh air to the deepest part of her lungs'. Hearing that, I was flooded with joyful feelings. I felt my heart expanding.

I asked Joy to whisper to the body again that ...she was about to wake up in a new healthy body. The operation was successful. The doctors had removed all possible sources of pain and had given her a new skin with extra strength inside. She was now in a new environment surrounded with love, and she would have lots of space to move around, to live her life, and to be herself. Joy seemed to be overjoyed while she was saying these wonderful words to this patient. Then we told the body to wake up when we counted to three.

'One...two...three...', I counted. Joy looked overwhelmed, with tears in her eyes. The splitting was over. The healer became one with the patient. We left the room, leaving the scene and those roles behind. Joy said that she was having a rebirth experience. The painful sensations she had had before the operation were drastically reduced. She felt thankful and was excited to go home with these new perceptions of her body.

Joy was secure enough to share this experience with her mother. She was straight to the point, and she was honest about her own feelings. Joy did not want to be accusatory. She still loved her mother, and they were able to spend time together. She only wished to hear someone say sorry, and her wish was granted. The following morning, Joy told the group that 70 per cent of her chronic pains had diminished overnight!

It has now been about a month, and Joy has started searching for a way to balance her personal life with the time that she could give to her mother. She is also hoping for a love relationship, wishing it to happen in natural ways and not pushing the matter. She is setting boundaries in relationship and is becoming more relaxed and more settled, with lots of time for herself. Joy is focusing on reconstructing relationships and is less bothered by the pain.

My experience with Joy in this process is invaluable. I feel thankful to her for letting me walk her healing path and allowing me to turn part of the walk into a play that we could both enjoy. This experience convinced me even more of the power of imagination in creating healing metaphors. The playful part that resides in myself is no different from the playful quality within Joy. Despite being in a devastating state, she was able to slip into her imagination and play with me. I am beginning to believe in what Peter Levine (2005) said in his book *Healing Trauma* that '…most organisms have an innate capacity to rebound from threatening and stressful events' (2005, 1). Levine also mentioned the Four Noble Truths of Buddha's Teaching, with which I could not agree more. He says:

> 'The transformative power of suffering finds perhaps its clearest expression in the Four Noble Truths espoused by the Buddha. Though suffering and trauma are not identical, the Buddha's insight into the nature of suffering can provide a powerful mirror for examining the effects of trauma in your life. The Buddha's basic teaching offers guidance for healing our trauma and recovering a sense of wholeness'.
>
> (2005, 4)

In this case study, the whole process we saw is the reality of these Four Noble Truths coming into play. Here, I believe that Johanne Hamel allows somatic art therapy to meet Buddhist philosophy.

## Notes

1 CiiAT stands for Canadian International Institute of Art Therapy. CiiAT provides art therapy education internationally, including formal training in Thailand, Japan, and online training across the globe.
2 IPATT stands for International Program of Art Therapy in Thailand. Founded in 2011, the IPATT program is hosted by Art Therapy Charitable Foundation in Thailand and is operated in conjunction with CiiAT.
3 The four Noble Truths in Buddhism comprises Dukkha, Samudaya, Nirodha, and Magga. Dukkha is the truth of suffering. Buddhist philosophy conceives suffering as part of human condition. Life without suffering does not exist. Samudaya is the truth of the origin of suffering. The origin of suffering can be the thirst for pleasure or power, a desire for immortality, etc. Nirodha is the truth of the cessation of suffering, a complete stopping, or a release from sorrow. Magga is the truth of the path leading to the cessation of suffering.

# Conclusion

## The Importance of Developing Somatic Art Therapy Research

*Johanne Hamel*

It is generally known that research in art therapy is not yet developed enough. There is a body of knowledge based on qualitative research (including clinical findings, case studies, research on diagnostic tools), but there is still too little. With respect to quantitative research in art therapy, it is almost non-existent. This is no surprise, considering that it is known that clinical practices often move forward by trial and error. In the USA, art therapy is recognized for the treatment of post-traumatic stress disorder (PTSD). However, it would be appropriate to validate our knowledge on PTSD and chronic pain by doing research that would be in line with the work of other scholars. As there are many avenues for research, an exhaustive list was not made here.

I would like to highlight one that seems of particular interest for chronic pain: the application of the SIBAM (sensation, image, behaviour, affect, and meaning) model to art therapy. This model seems very effective; it reflects many of my clinical findings, as I found out that paying attention to one element of the model gives access to the others. It would be interesting to flesh out the *power of images* that gives access to the dissociated elements and reconnects the right brain and the left brain, and to demonstrate through research how it could be used in art therapy without re-traumatizing the client.

As a research avenue, Bessel van der Kolk suggests checking whether attaching semantic representations to trauma (putting words to it), which art therapy seems to do by reconnecting the right brain and the left brain, would effectively reduce amygdala activation and sensory associations during exposure to trauma memories. Demonstrating this in art therapy would formally support the effectiveness of this approach.

Developing the somatic art therapy approach, supported by our understanding of the emotional memory reconsolidation that it allows, is of particular interest to art therapy as well. Rothschild's (2000) and van der Kolk's perceptions support the use of the somatic memory for treating trauma:

'Using the body itself as a potential resource to treat trauma has rarely been explored. Somatic memory has been recognized as a phenomenon but few scientifically supported strategies and theories have emerged to recognize it and use it in the therapeutic process'.[1]

I would like to conclude by citing the following statement from Bessel van der Kolk:

'While it is true that at the heart of the incoherence affecting traumatized and neglected patients lies the problem of being unable to analyze what is occurring when they re-experience the physical sensations of past traumas - and these sensations produce intense emotions that cannot be modulated-, it means that therapy must serve the purpose of helping patients stay in their bodies and understand their bodily sensations. And it's certainly not something that conventional therapies, which we have all been taught, can successfully help people do'.[2]

Finally, art therapy and especially somatic art therapy, supported by the quantum model, offer new promising perspectives for the treatment of PTSD and chronic pain. As various states of consciousness are shown to have a crucial influence in the manifestation of disease and health, developing the research in the quantum field framework can provide professional art therapists with a unique tool to teach their clients how to release ego-based consciousness, allowing them to use somatic art therapy as a bridge towards unity consciousness and healing.

## Notes

1  Bessel van der Kolk,1998, in Rothschild, B. (2000): *Op. Cit.* 5.
2  Bessel van der Kolk,1998, in Rothschild, B. (2000): *Op. Cit.* 3.

# Appendices

# Appendix A

## Diagnostic criteria of PTSD (DSM V, 2013)[1]

Note: The following criteria apply to adults, adolescents and children older than 6 years. For children 6 years and younger, see corresponding criteria below.

A. Exposure to actual or threatened death, serious injury, or sexual violence in one (or more) of the following ways:

1 Directly experiencing the traumatic event(s).
2 Witnessing, in person, the event(s) as it occurred to others.
3 Learning that the traumatic event(s) occurred to a close family member or close friend. In cases of actual or threatened death of a family member or friend, the event(s) must have been violent or accidental.
4 Experiencing repeated or extreme exposure to aversive details of the traumatic event(s) (e.g., first responders collecting human remains; police officers repeatedly exposed to details of child abuse).

Note: Criterion A4 does not apply to exposure through electronic media, television, movies, or pictures, unless this exposure is work-related.

B. Presence of one (or more) of the following intrusion symptoms associated with the traumatic event(s), beginning after the traumatic event(s) occurred:

1 Recurrent, involuntary, and intrusive distressing memories of the traumatic event(s)

Note: In children older than six years, repetitive play can occur in which themes or aspects of the traumatic event(s) are expressed.

2 Recurring distressing dreams in which the content and/or effect of the dream are related to the traumatic event(s).

Note: In children, there could be frightening dreams without recognizable content.

3   Dissociative reactions (e.g., flashbacks) in which the individual feels or acts as if the traumatic event(s) were recurring. (Such reactions might occur on a continuum, with the most extreme expression being a complete loss of awareness of present surroundings.)

Note: In children, trauma-specific re-enactment can occur in play.

4   Intense or prolonged psychological distress at exposure to internal or external cues that symbolize or resemble an aspect of the traumatic event(s).
5   Marked physiological reactions to internal or external cues that symbolize or resemble an aspect of the traumatic event(s).

C. Persistent avoidance of stimuli associated with the traumatic event(s), beginning after the traumatic event(s) occurred, as evidenced by one or both of the following:

1   Avoidance of or efforts to avoid distressing memories, thoughts, or feelings about or closely associated with the traumatic event(s).
2   Avoidance of or efforts to avoid external reminders (people, places, conversations, activities, objects, situations) that arouse distressing memories, thoughts, or feelings about or closely associated with the traumatic event(s).

D. Negative alterations in cognitions and mood associated with the traumatic event(s), beginning or worsening after the traumatic event(s) occurred, as evidenced by two (or more) of the following:

1   Inability to remember an important aspect of the traumatic event(s) (typically owing to dissociative amnesia and not to other factors such as head injury, alcohol, or drugs).
2   Persistent and exaggerated negative beliefs or expectations about oneself, others, or the world (e.g., 'I am bad', 'No one can be trusted', 'The world is completely dangerous', 'My whole nervous system is permanently ruined').
3   Persistent, distorted cognitions about the cause or consequences of the traumatic event(s) that cause the individual to blame himself/ herself or others.
4   Persistent negative emotional state (e.g., fear, horror, anger, guilt, or shame).
5   Markedly diminished interest or participation in significant activities.
6   Feelings of detachment or estrangement from others.

7   Persistent inability to experience positive emotions (e.g., inability to experience happiness, satisfaction, or loving feelings).

E. Marked alterations in arousal and reactivity associated with the traumatic event(s), beginning or worsening after the traumatic event(s) occurred, as evidenced by two (or more) of the following:

1   Irritable behavior and angry outbursts (with little or no provocation) typically expressed as verbal or physical aggression toward people or objects.
2   Reckless or self-destructive behavior.
3   Hypervigilance.
4   Exaggerated startle response.
5   Problems with concentration.
6   Sleep disturbance (e.g. difficulty falling or staying asleep or restless sleep).

F. Duration of the disturbance (Criteria B, C, D, and E) is more than one month.
G. The disturbance causes clinically significant distress or impairment in social, occupational, or other important areas of functioning.
H. The disturbance is not attributable to physiological effects of a substance (e.g., medication, alcohol) or another medical condition. Specify if:

**With dissociative symptoms:** the individual's symptoms meet the criteria for post-traumatic stress disorder, and in addition, in response to the stressor, the individual experiences persistent or recurrent symptoms of either of the following:

1   **Depersonalization**: Persistent or recurrent experiences of feeling detached from, and as if one were an outside observer of, one's mental processes or body (e.g., feeling as though one were in a dream; feeling a sense of unreality of self or body or of time moving slowly).
2   **Derealization**: Persistent or recurrent experiences of unreality of surroundings (e.g., the world around the individual is experienced as unreal, dreamlike, distant, or distorted).

Note: To use this subtype, the dissociative symptoms must not be attributable to the physiological effects of a substance (e.g., blackouts, behavior during alcohol intoxication) or another medical condition (e. g., complex partial seizures).

Specify if:
**With delayed expression**: If the full diagnostic criteria are not met until at least six months after the event (although the onset and expression of some symptoms might be immediate).

## Post-traumatic stress disorder for children aged six years and younger

A. In children aged six years and younger, exposure to actual or threatened death, serious injury, or sexual violence in one (or more) of the following ways:

1 Directly experiencing the traumatic event(s).
2 Witnessing, in person, the event(s) as it occurred to others, especially primary caregivers.

Note: Witnessing does not include events that are witnessed only in electronic media, television, movies, or pictures.

3 Learning that he traumatic event(s) occurred to a parent or caregiving figure.

B. Presence of one (or more) of the following intrusion symptoms associated with the traumatic event(s), beginning after he traumatic event(s) occurred:

1 Recurrent, involuntary, and intrusive distressing memories of the traumatic event(s).

Note: Spontaneous and intrusive memories might not necessarily appear distressing and might be expressed as play re-enactment.

2 Recurrent distressing dreams in which the content and/or effects of the dream are related to the traumatic event(s).

Note: It might not be possible to ascertain that the frightening content is related to the traumatic event.

3 Dissociative reactions (e.g., flashbacks) in which the child feels or acts as if the traumatic event(s) were recurring. (Such reactions might occur on a continuum, with the most extreme expression being a complete loss of awareness of present surroundings.) Such trauma-specific re-enactment might occur in play.
4 Intense or prolonged psychological distress at exposure to internal or external cues that symbolize or resemble an aspect of the traumatic event(s).
5 Marked physiological reactions to reminders of the traumatic event(s).

C. One (or more) of the following symptoms, representing either persistent avoidance of stimuli associated with the traumatic event(s) or negative alterations in cognitions and mood associated with the traumatic event(s), must be present, beginning after the event(s) or worsening after the event(s):

Persistent avoidance of stimuli:

1    Avoidance of or efforts to avoid activities, places, or physical reminders that arouse recollections of the traumatic event(s).
2    Avoidance of or efforts to avoid people, conversations, or inter-personal situations that arouse recollections of the traumatic event(s).

Negative alterations in cognitions:

1    Substantially increased frequency of negative emotional state (e.g., fear, guilt, sadness, shame, confusion).
2    Markedly diminished interest or participation in significant activities, including constriction of play.
3    Socially withdrawn behavior.
4    Persistent reduction in expression of positive emotions.

D. Alterations in arousal and reactivity associated with the traumatic event(s), beginning or worsening after the traumatic event(s) occurred, as evidenced by two (or more) of the following:

1    Irritable behavior and angry outbursts (with little or no provocation) typically expressed as verbal or physical aggression toward people or objects (including extreme temper tantrums).
2    Hypervigilance.
3    Exaggerated startle response.
4    Problems with concentration.
5    Sleep disturbance (e.g. difficulty falling or staying asleep or restless sleep).

E. Duration of the disturbance is more than one month.
F. The disturbance causes clinically significant distress or impairment in relationships with parents, siblings, peers, or other caregivers or with school behavior.
G. The disturbance is not attributable to physiological effects of a substance (e.g., medication, alcohol) or another medical condition.

Specify if:
**With dissociative symptoms:** the individual's symptoms meet the criteria for posttraumatic stress disorder, and the individual experiences persistent or recurrent symptoms of either of the following:

1    **Depersonalization:** Persistent or recurrent experiences of feeling detached from, and as if one were an outside observer of, one's mental

processes or body (e.g., feeling as though one were in a dream; feeling a sense of unreality of self or body or of time moving slowly).

2  **Derealization**: Persistent or recurrent experiences of unreality of surroundings (e.g., the world around the individual is experienced as unreal, dreamlike, distant or distorted).

Note: To use this subtype, the dissociative symptoms must not be attributable to the physiological effects of a substance (e.g., blackouts) or another medical condition (e.g., complex partial seizures).

Specify if:
**With delayed expression**: If the full diagnostic criteria are not met until at least six months after the event (although the onset and expression of some symptoms might be immediate).

## Acute stress disorder

A. Exposure to actual or threatened death, serious injury, or sexual violence in one (or more) of the following ways:

1  Directly experiencing the traumatic event(s).
2  Witnessing, in person, the event(s) as it occurred to others.
3  Learning that the traumatic event(s) occurred to a close family member or close friend.

Note: In cases of actual or threatened death of a family member or friend, the event(s) must have been violent or accidental.

4  Experiencing repeated or extreme exposure to aversive details of the traumatic event(s) (e.g., first responders collecting human remains; police officers repeatedly exposed to details of child abuse).

Note: This does not apply to exposure through electronic media, television, movies or pictures, unless this exposure is work related.

B. Presence of nine (or more) of the following symptoms from any of the categories of intrusion, negative mood, dissociation, avoidance, and arousal, beginning or worsening after the traumatic event(s) occurred:

## Intrusion symptoms

1  Recurrent, involuntary, and intrusive distressing memories of the traumatic event(s).

Note: In children, repetitive play might occur in which themes or aspects of the traumatic event(s) are expressed.

2   Recurring distressing dreams in which the content and/or effect of the dream are related to the traumatic event(s).

Note: In children, there might be frightening dreams without recognizable content.

3   Dissociative reactions (e.g., flashbacks) in which the individual feels or acts as if the traumatic event(s) were recurring. (Such reactions might occur on a continuum, with the most extreme expression being a complete loss of awareness of present surroundings.)

Note: In children, trauma-specific re-enactment might occur in play.

4   Intense or prolonged psychological distress or marked physiological reactions in response to internal or external cues that symbolize or resemble an aspect of the traumatic event(s).

## Negative mood

1   Persistent inability to experience positive emotions (e.g., inability to experience happiness, satisfaction, or loving feelings).

## Dissociative symptoms

1   An altered sense of the reality of one's surroundings or oneself (e.g., seeing oneself from another's perspective, being in a daze, time slowing).
2   Inability to remember an important aspect of the traumatic event(s) (typically due to dissociative amnesia and not to other factors such as head injury, alcohol or drugs).

## Avoidance symptoms

1   Efforts to avoid distressing memories, thoughts, or feelings about or closely associated with the traumatic event(s).
2   Efforts to avoid external reminders (people, places, conversations, activities, objects, situations) that arouse distressing memories, thoughts, or feelings about or closely associated with the traumatic event(s).

## Arousal symptoms

1   Sleep disturbance (e.g. difficulty falling or staying asleep or restless sleep).
2   Irritable behavior and angry outbursts (with little or no provocation), typically expressed as verbal or physical aggression toward people or objects.

3    Hypervigilance.
4    Problems with concentration.
5    Exaggerated startle response.

C. Duration of the disturbance (Symptoms in criterion B) is three days to one month after trauma exposure.

Note: Symptoms typically begin immediately after the trauma but persistence for at least 3 days and up to a month is needed to meet disorder criteria.

D. The disturbance causes clinically significant distress or impairment in social, occupational, or other important areas of functioning.

E. The disturbance is not attributable to physiological effects of a substance (e.g., medication or alcohol) or another medical condition (e.g., mild traumatic brain injury) and is not better explained by brief psychotic disorder.

# Appendix B

## The Bowl of Light[2]

### *The legend*

'Once, a long time ago, there was this wonderful old grandma who lived on the tiny island of Moloka'i. Her name was Kaili'ohe Kame'ekua and she was over 100 years old when she died in 1931. Grandma Kame'ekua and her family taught the children by stories, ancient chants, and parables. One story that was *really* important to her 'ohana (which means 'family' in Hawai'ian), is that every child is born with *a bowl of perfect light*. If the child takes good care of the light, it will grow and become strong. The child will be able to do many things, such as swim with the sharks, and fly with birds, and the child will be able to know many things. However, sometimes there are negativities that come into a child's life..... There are hurts, angers, jealousies, or pain. And these hurts, angers, or pain become like stones that drop into the bowl. And pretty soon there might be so many stones you cannot see the light... and pretty soon the child can become like a stone, he or she cannot grow.... cannot move. You see, light and stone cannot hold the same space. But what Grandma Kame'ekua tells us is that all the child needs to do is turn the bowl upside down and empty the stones and the light will grow once more.... Yes, the light *is* always there'.[3]

After hearing about this legend, Joyce Mills began including the Bowl of Light as an exercise in her workshops. She felt that this exercise could 'help rebuild and enhance a sense of self-esteem and self-appreciation...'[4]. She used the Bowl of Light exercise in two different ways: by creating the Bowl of Light or by simply drawing the Bowl of Light.

## Creating the Bowl of Light

Mills suggested using fast-drying, self-hardening clay and decorating the Bowl with acrylic paints. I found that using some kind of modeling compound made of *papier-mâché* works very well too as it is also fast drying and you can paint on it even when it's still wet. Mills also suggested to decorate the Bowl with small objects gathered from nature or special ones that had significant meaning for the person doing his or her Bowl of

Light. The Bowl has to be done in two different moments, to allow time for the clay to dry if that is what you are using.

### Drawing the Bowl of Light

Mills also liked the idea of drawing a Bowl of light using a simple piece of paper, writing the words 'Bowl of Light' across the top, and simply decorating the Bowl with art materials and significant symbols.[5]

Of particular interest to me is a *therapeutic ritual* she suggested after the creation of the Bowl: *Identifying, gathering, and letting go of your stones.*

She suggested to identify every obstacle to your inner light; those could be beliefs about life, about yourself, about your capacity to reach your goals or about your personal value; they could also be negative events in your life that dampened your spirit. Then she says: Once identified, gather one stone for each obstacle. Next, ask your clients to take their time and decide how, when and where they want to let them go.[6]

It is important to be ready before letting them go. Many things might be at play here. So respect your own timing. Most importantly, as Mills stated, 'Letting go of stones doesn't mean that the incident or experience never happened, it just allows your client to reconnect to the light he or she was born with – the innate ability to appreciate the self'.[7]

I find it most useful when clients let go of stones which represent attitudes, beliefs or behaviors they developed following negative situations in their lives, when those are not helping them any more.

# Appendix C

## The 'four-quadrants' somatic art therapy method

The 'four-quadrants' method is said to be a somatic art therapy method because we work with the inner sensations of the person; the word 'soma' refers to the inner sensation whereas the word 'body' refers to the external reality of the person, as perceived by others.

The four-quadrants method is a sequence of four interrelated drawings or paintings, with specific themes for each of the four productions. Each of these themes and production has a specific purpose. The total experience frequently helps to alleviate acute or chronic pain.

The sequence is based on neurosciences so that each of the four productions contributes in a meaningful way to the healing of the specific physical pain chosen by a client.

Although the method is specifically designed to treat physical pain, we can also adapt that same sequence to emotional distress. Physical pain is always connected to emotional pain anyway. Dawson Church (2003), author of several books on the emotional freedom technique (EFT), also known as the 'tapping method', explains in his books that scientifically, 80 to 90 per cent of physical pain is actually emotional. If we can reduce the emotional pain associated with a specific physical pain, the residual pain is then no more than 10 to 20 per cent of what it was before treatment.

I usually refer to the four-quadrants method as the 'giant mandala method' because when space allows it, we draw the four productions in a large 1.50 m circle separated in four equal parts. When it is not possible, I will simply offer participants four large sheets of papers (18 x 24 inches or 45 x 60 cm), recreating the same sequence. The 1.50 m circle allows for a better sense of the connectedness of the four productions and of the total experience, simply because we can see them all at once. Also, the circle gives it meaning by creating a sense of security; it contains the total experience in its rounded form.

I will now explain each of the four productions of the sequence, their themes, and their purpose in the whole experience.

## The first quadrant: The sensation (on the top right part of the mandala)

For this first production, I ask my client to choose a painful sensation, in a specific part of the body. The instruction is to draw a current or often present physical pain, focusing specifically on the painful *sensation*. If the person does not know what sensation to choose or if she is not used to attend to her bodily sensations, I might first guide her through a meditation or relaxation centered on her inner sensations. I usually do such a meditation when working with a group.

Once the person has chosen a specific painful sensation, my first assignment will be to draw the contour of the body part on which the person wants to work. For instance, if she has a burning sensation in her right foot, I will ask her to draw first the contour of her right foot. Then, once it is done, I ask that she draws the physical sensation in that part of her body, for instance, the burning sensation.

The word 'sensation' here is key to somatic art therapy. For this method to work in the best way possible, the client needs to concentrate on the pure physical sensation itself, be it a burning sensation, a constriction, a throbbing, a tearing, whatever the sensation is, and to represent it as closely as possible with lines, forms, colors, and media. Often, the person will not understand why she is drawing or painting it in that specific way. It does not matter; the point is to observe closely this inner painful sensation, now contained on the paper. Once this is done, we are ready to work on the second quadrant, in the top left in the giant mandala.

## The second quadrant: The origin (in the top left of the giant mandala)

This time, my instruction to the client is to draw or paint the very first time he experienced that painful sensation. Most of the time, as soon as I give this suggestion, a specific image of a difficult moment of the past comes to mind: an inner tension, a traumatic moment, a psychological pain, a meaningful interpersonal moment.

I then ask the person to either draw the event itself, in a figurative way, or to draw how he/she felt at that moment. Sometimes, a person cannot find the very first time that pain was felt. So then I ask to draw an example of the type of situation in which the pain will manifest itself. I know that this situation will somehow be connected to the symbolic meaning of the pain.

Because pain *is a symbol*. Pain is *a dream of the body*, as Arnold Mindell (1985, 2014) explains in his books on the *dreambody approach*; it is a symbol which carries a meaning, a symbol that has something to say. In French, we have a saying: 'Les maux expriment ce que les mots n'ont pas su dire', which means that the body expresses what the words have not been able to say. With this second quadrant, we are trying to get to the original non-expressed emotional pain. And we find it most of the time.

Or we find a self-sabotaging behavior that the person reproduces unconsciously, a behavior that maintains emotional pain.

### The third production in the fourth quadrant: The healing (bottom right of the giant mandala)

We draw or paint the third drawing at the bottom right of the mandala, which is the fourth quadrant. Here, the instruction given is to draw again the contour of the same specific part of the body the person is working on, but this time, the person draws how that part would look like visually if the pain was totally gone and if it would feel totally good and even pleasurable. By doing that, the person creates an image allowing the psyche to develop a new neurological pathway in the limbic system, mostly in the right hemisphere of the brain. That image opens up new possibilities of well-being for the person. Time and again, people will immediately start to feel better and they will tell me that they now have hope that they can eventually live with less pain or even, eventually, without pain. That image is said to be 'implicit', as we cannot tell the body what to do exactly in his inner processes to create that wellbeing, but the psyche and the body understand that language and they will soon begin to change toward the new condition.

### The fourth production in the third quadrant: The transition quadrant (bottom left of the giant mandala)

The fourth drawing or painting is said to be the transition. Here we want to find concrete ways and actions in daily life in order to make the healing possible and to maintain it. Often, what is called for in this drawing is an expression of the emotions that were repressed at the time of the original event: sadness, emotional distress, anger, rage, disgust, despair, grief, whatever the painful emotion was. Other times, the person is able to see what behavior that she needs to change in order to prevent the re-occurring of the physical pain; for instance, to stop saying 'yes' when she actually means 'no', to walk away from a detrimental relationship, to learn affirmation skills, to change job, or whatever makes sense.

We have specific instructions to help find the transition if it is not already clear or evident for the client. We will suggest, for instance, to create a new drawing using lines, forms, colors of the first drawing (the pain), as well as lines, forms, and colors of the third drawing (the healing). While doing so, often a solution will appear in this sort of 'middle drawing'. This is the most difficult task of the four productions, and clients often need our help to identify the right transition. In this quadrant, we are working with the left side of the brain because we explicitly want to find a way to create the well-being: we plan actions, an attitude change, new behaviors, choices that we know need to be made. We are also working with the right side of the brain, or the implicit processes, because the transition will help to create new neurological pathways. We know from neurosciences that the more we repeat a new behavior, the more we create and solidify new pathways in the brain, because of the neuroplasticity of the brain: the brain is forever changing and adapting with each new experience.

## Notes

1  American Psychological Association (2013). *Mini-Desk reference to the DSM-V.* Washington, DC: APA, 143–151.
2  Mills, J. (2006). The Bowl of Light: A Story-Craft for Healing. In: Carey, L. (Ed.): *Expressive and Creative Methods for Trauma Survivors.* Philadelphia,PA: Jessica Kingsley, 207–213.
3  Mills, J. (2006). *Op. Cit.,* 208–209.
4  Mills, J. (2006), 210.
5  For more specific instructions, see Mills (2006), *idem,* 210–212.
6  Mills (2006), *idem,* p. 212.
7  Mills (2006), *idem,* p. 213.

# Bibliography

**References for art therapists**

*In English*

American Psychiatric Association. (2013). *Mini-Desk Reference to the Diagnostic Criteria from the DSM-V.* Washington, DC: American Psychological Association.

Asmundson, G. J. G., Coons, M. J., Taylor, S. & Katz, J. (2002). PTSD and the experience of pain: research and clinical implications of shared vulnerability and mutual maintenance models. *Canadian Journal of Psychiatry, 47*(10), 930–937.

Asmundson, G. J. G., Wright, K. D., McCreary, D. R. & Pedlar, D. (2003). Post-traumatic stress disorder symptoms in United Nations peacekeepers with and without chronic pain. *Cognitive Behavior Therapy, 32*(1), 26–37.

Camic, P. M. (1999). Expanding treatment possibilities for chronic pain through the expressive arts. In: Malchiodi, C. (Ed.) (1999). *Medical Art Therapy with Adults.* Philadelphia, PA: Jessica Kingsley.

Carey, L. (2006). *Expressive and Creative Arts Methods for Trauma Survivors.* London and Philadelphia, PA: Jessica Kingsley.

Chesner, A. & Lykou, S. (2020). *Trauma in the Creative and Embodied Therapies: When Words Are Not Enough.* New York, NY and London: Routledge.

Cozolino, (2016). *Why Therapy Works. Using Our Brains To Change Our Minds.* New York, NY and London: W.W. Norton & Company.

Engle, P. (1997). Art therapy and dissociative disorders. *Art Therapy, Journal of the American Art Therapy Association, 14*(4), 246–254.

Hass-Cohen, N. & Findlay, J. C. (2015). *Art Therapy & The Neuroscience of Relationship, Creativity & Resiliency. Skills and Practices.* New York, NY: W. W. Norton & Company.

Hass-Cohen, N. & Findlay, J. C. (2019). The art therapy relational neuroscience and memory reconsolidation four drawing protocol. *The Arts in Psychotherapy, 63*, 51–59.

Hinz, L. (2009). *Expressive Therapies Continuum. A Framework For Using Art In Therapy.* New York, NY: Routledge.

Jacobson, M. (1994). Abreacting and assimilating traumatic, dissociated memories of MPD patients through art therapy. *Art Therapy, Journal of the American Art Therapy Association, 11*(1), 48–52.

Johnson, D. R. (1987). Perspective: The role of the creative arts therapies in the diagnosis and treatment of psychological trauma. *The Arts in Psychotherapy, An International Journal, 14*(1), 7–14.

Levine, P. (2015). *Trauma and Memory. Brain and Body in Search for the Living Past. A Practical Guide for Understanding and Working with Traumatic Memory.* Berkeley, CA: North Atlantic Books.

Levine, P. (2009). *Trauma, Tragedy, Therapy. The Arts and Human Suffering.* London and Philadelphia, PA: Jessica Kingsley.

Levine, P. A. (2005). *Healing Trauma, A Pioneering Program for Restoring the Wisdom of Your Body.* Korea: Sounds True.

Levine, P. (1997). *Waking the Tiger.* Berkeley, CA: North Atlantic Press.

Lindy, J. D., Green, B. L., Grace, M. (1992). Somatic reenactment in the treatment of posttraumatic stress disorder. *Psychotherapy and Psychosomatics, 57,* 180–186.

Malchiodi, C. (Ed.) (1999). *Medical Art Therapy with Adults.* Philadelphia, PA: Jessica Kingsley.

Malchiodi, C. (2020). *Trauma and Expressive Arts Therapy: Brain, Body, and Imagination in the Healing Process.* New York and London: Guilford Press.

Morgan III, C. A. & Johnson, D. R. (1995). Use of a drawing task in the treatment of nightmares in combat-related post-traumatic stress disorder. *Art Therapy, 12*(4), 244–247.

Otis, J. D., Keane, T. M. & Kerns, R. D. (2003). An examination of the relationship between chronic pain and post-traumatic stress disorder. *Journal of Rehabilitation Research and Development, 40*(5), 397–406.

Rothschild, B. (2000). *Body Remembers. The Psychophysiology of Trauma and Trauma Treatment.* New York, NY: W.W. Norton & Company.

Rhinehart, L. & Engelhorn, P. (1984). The full rainbow-Symbol of individuation. *The Arts in Psychotherapy, 11,* 37–43.

Scaer, R. C. (2001). *The Body Bears the Burden. Trauma, Dissociation, and Disease.* Binghamton, NY: The Haworth Medical Press.

Schnyder, U. & Cloitre, M. (2015). *Evidence-based Treatments for Trauma-related Psychological Disorders: A Practical Guide for Clinicians.* Cham: Springer.

Van der Kolk, B. A. (1987). *Psychological Trauma.* Washington, DC: American Psychiatric Press.

Van der Kolk, B. A. (1994). The body keeps the score. *Review of Psychiatry, 1,* 253–265.

Van der Kolk, B. A. (1996). The body keeps the score: approaches to the psychobiology of posttraumatic stress disorder. In: Van der Kolk, B. A., McFarlane, A. C. & Weisaeth, L., (1996). *Traumatic Stress: The Effects of Overwhelming Experience on Mind, Body, and Society,* 214–241. New York, NY: Guilford Press.


*In French*

Brillon, P. (2017b). *Comment aider les victimes souffrant de stress post-traumatique. Guide à l'intention des thérapeutes.* Montréal, QC: Québec-Livres.

Hamel, J. (2001). La psychothérapie par l'art: la transformation intérieure par la voie de l'imaginaire. *Revue Québécoise de Psychologie, 22*(1), 33–48.

Heusch, N. & Shermarke, M. (2001). Art-thérapie et reconstruction identitaire: Dévoilement d'expériences traumatiques dans un groupe de femmes réfugiées. *Prisme, 35,* 52–70.

Lambert, J. & Simard, P. (1997). L'art-thérapie, approche auprès des femmes adultes victimes d'agression à caractère sexuel durant l'enfance ou l'adolescence. *Revue Québécoise de Psychologie, 18*(3), 203–228.

Rinfret, M. (2000). Intégration des écoutes psychologiques et somatiques. *Revue Québécoise de Psychologie, 21(*1), 39–56.

### References for traumatized persons

#### *In English*

Carey, L. (2006). *Expressive and Creative Arts Methods for Trauma Survivors.* London and Philadelphia, PA: Jessica Kingsley.

Johnson, E. (2020). *Finding Comfort During Hard Times: A Guide to Healing After Disaster, Violence, and Other Community Trauma.* Lanham, MD: Rowman & Littlefield.

Levine, P. (1997). *Waking the Tiger.* Berkeley, CA: North Atlantic Press.

Rothschild, B. (2000). *Body Remembers. The Psychophysiology of Trauma and Trauma Treatment.* New York, NY: W. W. Norton & Company.

Scaer, R. C. (2001). *The Body Bears the Burden. Trauma, Dissociation, and Disease.* Binghamton, NY: The Haworth Medical Press.

Turk, D. C. & Winter, F. (2020). *The Pain Survival Guide: How to Become Resilient and Reclaim Your Life.* Washington, DC: American Psychological Association.

Van der Kolk, B. A. (1996). The body keeps the score: approaches to the psychobiology of posttraumatic stress disorder. In: Van der Kolk, B. A., McFarlane, A. C. & Weisaeth, L., (1996). *Traumatic Stress: the Effects of Overwhelming Experience on Mind, Body, and Society,* 214–241. New York, NY: Guilford Press.

#### *In French*

Association québécoise de la douleur chronique. (2006). Composer avec la douleur chronique. Published in Québec newspapers.

Beauchamp, Y. (2019). Le soulagement de la douleur: aspect médical. *Frontières,* (online periodical), *8*(2), 32–34. Available at: http://repere3.sdm.qc.ca/cgi-bin/rep texte.cgi?9660271 +logo (Accessed September 28, 2019).

Brillon, P. (2017). *Se Relever d'un Traumatisme: Réapprendre à Vivre et à Faire Confiance.* Montréal, QC: Québec-Livres.

Duchastel, A. (2005). *La Voie de l'Imaginaire. Le Processus en Art-thérapie.* Montréal, QC: Québec-Livres.

Hamel, J. (2001). La psychothérapie par l'art: la transformation intérieure par la voie de l'imaginaire. *Revue Québécoise de Psychologie, 22*(1), 33–48.

Jobin, A.-M. (2002/2020). *Le nouveau journal créatif.*Montréal, QC: Édition de l'Homme.

Jobin, A-M. (2013). *Créer la Vie qui vous Ressemble.* Montréal, QC: Le Jour.

Lambert, J. & Simard, P. (1997). L'art-thérapie, approche auprès des femmes adultes victimes d'agression à caractère sexuel durant l'enfance ou l'adolescence. *Revue Québécoise de Psychologie, 18*(3), 203–228.

### General bibliography

Achterberg, J. (1985). *Imagery in Healing. Shamanism and Modern Medicine.* Boulder, CO: Shambhala Publications.

American Psychiatric Association. (2013). *Mini-Desk Reference to the Diagnostic Criteria from the DSM-V.* Washington, DC: American Psychiatric Association.

Anderson, F. E. (1995). Catharsis and empowerment through group clay work with incest survivors. *The Arts in Psychotherapy, 22*(5), 413–427.

Asmundson, G. J. G., Wright, K. D., McCreary, D. R. & Pedlar, D. (2003). Post-traumatic stress disorder symptoms in United Nations peacekeepers with and without chronic pain. *Cognitive Behavior Therapy, 32*(1), 6–37.

Asmundson, G. J. G., Coons, M. J., Taylor, S. & Katz, J. (2002). PTSD and the experience of pain: research and clinical implications of shared vulnerability and mutual maintenance models. *Canadian Journal of Psychiatry, 47*(10), 930–937.

Association Québécoise de la Douleur |Chronique. (2006). *Composer avec la douleur chronique.* Published in Québec newspapers.

Baker, B. A. (2005). Art speaks in healing survivors of war: The use of art therapy in treating trauma survivors. *Journal of Aggression, Maltreatment and Trauma, 12*(1/2), 183–198.

Beauchamp, Y. (1995). Le soulagement de la douleur: aspect médical. *Frontières* (online periodical), *8*(2) 32–34.

Beckham, J. C., Crawford, A. L., Feldman, M. E., Kirby, A.C., Hertzberg, M.A., Davidson, R. J. T. & Moore, S. (1997). Chronic post-traumatic stress disorder and chronic pain in Vietnam combat veterans. *Journal of Psychosomatic Resources, 43*, 379–389.

Benedikt, R. A. & Kolb, L. C. (1986). Preliminary findings on chronic pain and posttraumatic stress disorder. *American Journal of Psychiatry, 143*, 908–910.

Berkowitz, S. (1990). Art therapy with a Vietnam veteran who has post-traumatic stress disorder. *Pratt Institute Creative Arts Therapy Review, 11*, 47–62.

Bonin, M., Norton, G. R., Frombach, I. & Asmundson, G. J. G. (2000). PTSD in different treatment settings: a preliminary investigation of PTSD symptomatology in substance abuse and chronic pain patients. *Depression and Anxiety, 11*, 131–133.

Brillon, P. (2017a). *Se Relever d'un Traumatisme: Réapprendre à Vivre et à Faire Confiance.* Montréal, QC: Québec-Livres.

Brillon. P. (2017b). *Comment Aider les Victimes Souffrant de Stress Post-traumatique: Guide à l'Intention des Thérapeutes.* Montréal, QC: Québec-Livres.

Brunet, A., Orr, S. P, Tremblay, J., Robertson, K., Nader, K. & Pitman, R. K. (2008). Effect of post-retrieval propranolol on psychophysiologic responding during subsequent script-driven traumatic imagery in post-traumatic stress disorder. *Journal of Psychiatric Research, 42*(6), 503–506.

Buchwald, D., Golderg, J., Noonans, C., Beals, J., Manson, S. & AI-SUPERPFP TEAM. (2005). Relationship between post-traumatic stress disorder and pain in two American Indian tribes. *Pain Medicine, 6*(1), 72–79.

Bryant, R. A., Marosszeky, J. E., Crooks, J., Baguley, I. J. & Gurba, J. A. (1999). Interaction of posttraumatic stress disorder and chronic pain following traumatic brain injury. *Journal of Head Trauma Rehabilitation, 14*(6), 588–591.

Camic, P. M. (1999). Expanding treatment possibilities for chronic pain through the expressive arts. In: Malchiodi, C. (Ed.) (1999). *Medical Art Therapy with Adults.* Philadelphia, PA: Jessica Kingsley.

Carey, L. (2006). *Expressive and Creative Arts Methods for Trauma Survivors.* London and Philadelphia, PA: Jessica Kingsley.

Case, C. (2005). *Imagining Animals: Art, Psychotherapy and Primitive States of Mind.* New York, NY: Routledge.

Chapman, L. (2014). *Neurobiologically-informed Trauma Therapy for Children and Adolescents: Understanding Mechanisms of Change*. New York, NY and London: W. W. Norton & Company.

Chesner, A. & Lykou, S. (2020). *Trauma in the Creative and Embodied Therapies: When Words Are Not Enough*. New York, NY and London: Routledge.

Chopra, D. (2009). *Reinventing the Body, Resurrecting the Soul*. New York, NY: Harmony Books.

Chopra, D. (2015). *Quantum Healing. Exploring the Frontiers of Mind/Body Medicine*. New York, NY: Penguin Random House.

Chopra, D. (2019). *Metahuman: Unleashing Your Infinite Potential*. New York, NY: Harmony Books.

Church, D. (2013). *The EFT Manual*. Santa Rosa, CA: Energy Psychology Press.

Church, D. (2018). *Clinical EFT Handbook. A Definitive Resource for Practitioners, Scholars, Clinicians and Researchers*. Santa Rosa, CA: Energy Psychology Press.

Ciano-Federoff, L. M. & Sperry, J. A. (2005). On "Converting" hand pain into psychological pain: treating hand pain vicariously through exposure-based therapy for PTSD. *Clinical Case Studies*, *4*(1), 57–71.

Cloitre, M. (1997). Somatic symptoms associated with PTSD: assessment and intervention. *NCP Clinical Quarterly* (online periodical), *7*(4).

Coan, J., Dchaefer, H. & Davidson, R. (2016). Lending a Hand: Social Regulation of the Neural Response to Threat. In Lipton, B. (Ed.). *Biology of Beliefs*. 161–162. Carlsbad, CA: Hay House.

Cohen, B., Barnes, M-M. & Rankin, A. B. (1995). *Managing Traumatic Stress Through Art: Drawing from the Center*. Derwood, MD: Sidran Press.

Cox, C. T., Cohen, B., Mills, B. & Sobol, B. (1991). Art by abuse survivors: A life cycle. In: *Image and Metaphor, the Practice and Profession of Art Therapy*. Mundelein, IL: American Art Therapy Association.

Cozolino, (2016). *Why Therapy Works. Using our Brains to Change Our Minds*. New York, NY and London: W.W. Norton & Company.

Deykin, E. Y., Keane, T. M., Kaloukep, D., Fincke, G., Rothendler, J., Siegfried, M. & Creamer, K. (2001). Posttraumatic stress disorder and the use of health services. *Psychosomatic Medicine*, *63*, 835–841.

Deyo, R. A., Cherkin, D., Conrad, D. & Volinn, E. (1991). Cost, controversy, crisis: Low back pain and the health of the public. *Annual Review of Public Health*, *12*, 41–156.

Duchastel, A. (2005). *La Voie de l'Imaginaire. Le Processus en Art-thérapie*. Montréal, QC: Quebecor.

Ecker, B., Ticic, R. & Hulley, L. (2012). *Unlocking the Emotional Brain. Eliminating Symptoms at their Roots Using Memory Reconsolidation*. New York, NY: Routledge.

Engle, P. (1997). Art therapy and dissociative disorders. *Art Therapy, Journal of the American Art Therapy Association*, *14*(4), 246–254.

Estep, M. (1995). To soothe oneself: Art therapy with a woman recovering from incest. *American Journal of Art Therapy*, *34*(1), 9–18.

Feinstein, D., Eden, D. & Craig, G. (2005). *The Promise of Energy Psychology: Revolutionary Tools for Dramatic Personal Change*. New York, NY: Jeremy P. Tarcher/Penguin.

Frey, D. (2006). Puppetry interventions for traumatized clients. In: Carey, L. (Ed.). *Expressive and Creative Arts Methods for Trauma Survivors*. London and Philadelphia, PA: Jessica Kingsley.

Friedman, M. J. & Schnurr, P. (1996). Trauma, PTSD, and Health. *NCP Clinical Quarterly* (online periodical), *6*(4).

Gazzaniga, M. S., Ivry, R. B. & Mangun, G. R. (2014). *Cognitive Neuroscience. The Biology of the Mind*. New York and London: W. W. Norton & Company.

Gebhart, R. J. & Neeley, F. L. (1996). Primary care and PTSD. *NCP Clinical Quarterly* (online periodical) *6(*4).

Glaister, J. A. (2000). Four years later: Clara Revisited. *Perspectives in Psychiatric Care, 36*(1), 5–13.

Gold, E. & Zahm, S. (2018). *Buddhist psychology and Gestalt Therapy Integrated. Psychotherapy for the 21st Century*. Metta Press (Kindle edition).

Golub, D. (1985). Symbolic expression in post-traumatic stress disorder: Vietnam combat veterans in art-therapy. *The Arts in Psychotherapy, An International Journal, 12*(4), 285–296.

Goswami, A. (2013). *Le Médecin Quantique*. Varennes, QC: ADA.

Grande, L. A., Loeser, J. D., Ozuna, J., Ashleigh, A. & Samii, A. (2004). Complex regional pain syndrome as a stress response. *Pain* (online periodical), *110*(1–2), 495–498.

Grant, M. & Threlfo, C. (2002). EMDR in the treatment of chronic pain. *Journal of clinical psychology* (online periodical), *58*(12), 1505–1520.

Greece, M. (2003). Art therapy on a bone marrow transplant unit: the case study of a Vietnam veteran fighting myelofibrosis. *The Arts in Psychotherapy, An International Journal, 30*(4), 229–238.

Guay, S. & Marchand, A. (2006). *Les Troubles Liés aux Evénements Traumatiques. Dépistage, Evaluation et Traitements*. Montréal, QC: Les Presses de l'Université de Montréal.

Hamel, J. (1997). L'approche gestaltiste en thérapie par l'art. *Revue Québécoise de Gestalt, 2*(1), 130–147.

Hamel, J. (2001). La psychothérapie par l'art: la transformation intérieure par la voie de l'imaginaire. *Revue Québécoise de Psychologie, 22*(1), 33–48.

Hamel, J. (2008). *Les Neurosciences et l'Art-thérapie*. (Unpublished). Sherbrooke, QC: Université de Sherbrooke.

Hamel, J. (2014). *L'Art-thérapie Somatique. Pour Aider à Guérir la Douleur Chronique*. 3rd Ed. Montréal, QC: Québec-Livres.

Hargrave-Nykaza, K. (1994). An application of art therapy to the trauma of rape. *Art therapy, Journal of the American Art Therapy Association, 11*(1), 53–57.

Hass-Cohen, N. & Findlay, J. C. (2019). The art therapy relational neuroscience and memory reconsolidation four drawing protocol. *The Arts in Psychotherapy, 63*, 51–59.

Hass-Cohen, N. & Findlay, J. C. (2015). *Art Therapy & the Neuroscience of Relationship, Creativity & Resiliency. Skills and Practices*. New York, NY: W. W. Norton & Company.

Hass-Cohen, N. & Carr, R. (2008). *Art Therapy and Clinical Neuroscience*. New York, NY and Philadelphia, PA: Jessica Kingsley.

HeartMath Institute. (2020). www.heartmath.org/research/science-of-the-heart. Accessed August 6, 2020.

Heusch, N. & Shermarke, M. (2001). Art-thérapie et reconstruction identitaire: Dévoilement d'expériences traumatiques dans un groupe de femmes réfugiées. *Prisme, 35,* 52–70.

Hines-Martin, V. P. & Ising, M. (1993). Use of art therapy with post-traumatic stress disordered veteran clients. *Journal of Psychosocial Nursing and Mental Health Services, 31*(9), 29–36.

Hinz, L. (2009). *Expressive Therapies Continuum. A Framework for Using Art in Therapy.* New York, NY: Routledge.

Howard, R. (1990). Art therapy as an isomorphic intervention in the treatment of a client with post-traumatic stress disorder. *The American Journal of Art Therapy, 28*(3), 79–87.

Jacobson, M. (1994). Abreacting and assimilating traumatic, dissociated memories of MPD patients through art therapy. *Art Therapy, Journal of the American Art Therapy Association, 11*(1), 48–52.

Jensen, M. P., Romano, J. M., Turner, J. A., Good, A. B. & Wald, L. H. (1999). Patient beliefs predict patient functioning: Further support for a cognitive-behavioral model of chronic pain. *Pain, 81,* 95–104.

Jobin, A-M. (2013). *Créer La Vie Qui Vous Ressemble.* Montréal, QC: Le Jour.

Jobin, A-M. (2002). *Le Journal Créatif. à la Rencontre de Soi par l'Art et l'Ecriture.* Montréal, QC: Éditions du Roseau.

Johnson, D. R. (1987). Perspective: The role of the creative arts therapies in the diagnosis and treatment of psychological trauma. *The Arts in Psychotherapy, An International Journal, 14*(1), 7–14.

Johnson, E. (2020). *Finding Comfort During Hard Times: A Guide To Healing After Disaster, Violence, And Other Community Trauma.* Lanham, MD: Rowman & Littlefield.

Jones, J. G. (1997). Art therapy with a community of survivors. *Art Therapy, Journal of the American Art Therapy Association, 14*(2), 89–94.

Jung, C. (1993). *La Guérison Psychologique.* Geneva: Éditions Georg.

Kluft, R. P. (1984). Aspects of the treatment of multiple personality disorder. *Psychiatric Annals, 14*(1), 51–55.

Knight, S. J. & Camic, P. M. (1998). Health psychology and medicine: The art and science of healing. In: Camic, P. M., Knight, S. J. (Eds). *Clinical handbook of health-psychology.* Seattle and Toronto, ON: Hogrefe & Huber.

Korn, D. L. & Leeds, A. M. (2002). Preliminary evidence of efficacy for EMDR resource development and installation in the stabilization phase of treatment of complex posttraumatic stress disorder. *Journal of Clinical psychology, 58*(12), 1465–1487.

Lacroix, L. (2002). Retour au pays d'origine. Créativité sensorielle par l'utilisation du jeu de sable en art-thérapie. *Prisme* (online periodical), *37,* 32–35.

Lambert, J. & Simard, P. (1997). L'art-thérapie, approche auprès des femmes adultes victimes d'agression à caractère sexuel durant l'enfance ou l'adolescence. *Revue Québécoise de Psychologie, 18*(3), 203–228.

Lang, P. J. (1979). A bioinformational theory of emotional imagery. *Psychophysiology, 52,* 1048–1060.

Lauterbach, D., Vora, R. & Rakow, M. (2005). The relationship between post-traumatic stress disorder and self-reported health problems. *Psychosomatic medicine* (online periodical), *67*(6).

LeDoux, J. (2015). *Anxious. The Modern Mind in the Age of Anxiety.* London: Oneworld.

Levine, P. A. (2015). *Trauma and Memory. Brain and Body in Search for the Living Past. A Practical Guide for Understanding and Working with Traumatic Memory.* Berkeley, CA: North Atlantic Books.

Levine, P. A. (2009). *Trauma, Tragedy, Therapy. The Arts and Human Suffering.* London and Philadelphia, PA: Jessica Kingsley.

Levine, P. A. (2008). *Healing Trauma, A Pioneering Program for Restoring the Wisdom of Your Body.* Korea: Sounds True.

Levine, P. A. (1997). *Waking the Tiger.* Berkeley, CA: North Atlantic Press.

Lev-Wiesel (1998). Use of a drawing technique to encourage verbalization in adult survivor of sexual abuse. *The Arts in Psychotherapy, 25*(4), 257–262.

Lewis, D. J. (1979). Psychobiology of active and inactive memory. *Psychological Bulletin, 86,* 1054–1083.

Lindy, J. D., Green, B. L. & Grace, M. (1992). Somatic re-enactment in the treatment of posttraumatic stress disorder. *Psychotherapy and Psychosomatics, 57,* 180–186.

Lipton, B. (2016). *Biology of Beliefs.* Carlsbad, CA: Hay House.

Lusebrink, V. B. (2004). Art therapy and the brain: an attempt to understand the underlying processes of art expression in therapy. *Art Therapy, Journal of the American Art Therapy Association, 24*(1), 125–135.

Lusebrink, V. B. (2014). Art therapy and the neural basis of imagery: another possible view. *Art Therapy, 31*(2), 87–90.

Malchiodi, C. (Ed.) (1999). *Medical Art Therapy with Adults.* Philadelphia, PA: Jessica Kingsley.

Malchiodi, C. (2020). *Trauma and Expressive Arts Therapy: Brain, Body, and Imagination in the Healing Process.* New York, NY and London: Guilford Press.

Mapp, I. & Koch, D. (2004). Creation of a group mural to promote healing following a mass trauma. In: Webb, N. B. (Ed.). *Mass trauma and violence: Helping families and children cope,* 100–119. New York, NY: Guilford Press.

Martin, E. (1997). The symbolic graphic life-line: integrating the past and present through graphic imagery. *Art Therapy, Journal of the American Art Therapy Association, 14*(4), 261–267.

Masquelier-Savatier, C. (2017). *La Gestalt-thérapie.* 2 ed. Paris: Presses Universitaires de France.

McCarthy, D. (2006). Sandplay therapy and the body in trauma recovery. In: Carey, L. (Ed.). *Expressive and Creative Arts Methods for Trauma Survivors.* London and Philadelphia, PA: Jessica Kingsley.

McFarlan, A. C., Atchison, M., Rafalowicz, E. & Papay, P. (1994). Physiological symptoms in posttraumatic stress disorder. *J Pychosom Res, 42,* 607–617.

McNiff, S. (1992). *Art as Medicine, Creating a Therapy of the Imagination.* Boston, MA: Shambhala Publications.

Melzack, R. M. (1996). Gate control theory: On the evolution of pain concepts. Pain Forum, *5,* 128–138.

Melzack, R. M. & Wall, P. D. (1965). Pain mechanisms: A new theory. *Science, 150,* 971–979.

Merriam, B. (1998). To find a voice: art therapy in a woman's prison. *Women and Therapy, 21*(1), 57–171.

Mills, J. (2006). The bowl of light: A story-craft for healing. In: Carey, L. (Ed.). *Expressive and Creative Arts Methods for Trauma Survivors*, 207–213. London and Philadelphia, PA: Jessica Kingsley.

Mindell, A. (1985). *River's Way. The Process Science of the Dreambody*. London: Arkana.

Mindell, A. (2014). *Working with the Dreaming Body*. 2 ed. Portland, OR: Lao Tse Press.

Modell, A. H. (2003). *Imagination and the Meaningful Brain*. Cambridge, MA: The MIT Press.

Morgan III, C. A. & Johnson, D. R. (1995). Use of a drawing task in the treatment of nightmares in combat-related post-traumatic stress disorder. *Art Therapy, 12* (4), 244–247.

Moorjani, A. (2014). *Vivre Pour Mourir: d'Une Expérience de Mort Imminente à la Complète Guérison du Cancer*. Québec, QC: Le Dauphin Blanc.

Mowrer, O. H. (1960). *Learning Theory and Behavior*. New York, NY: Wiley.

Muraoka, M., Komiyama, H., Hosoi, M., Mine, K. & Kubo, C. (1996). Psychosomatic treatment of phantom limb pain with post-traumatic stress disorder. *Pain, 66*(2–3), 385–388.

Muse, M. (1986). Stress-related, posttraumatic chronic pain syndrome: behavioral treatment approach. *Pain, 25*, 389–394.

Nader, K., Schafe, G. E. & Le Doux, J. E. (2000). Fear memories require protein synthesis in the amygdala for reconsolidation after retrieval. *Nature, 406*, 722–726.

Naparastek, B. (2004). *Invisible Heroes. Survivors of Trauma and How They Heal*. New York, NY: Bantam Dell.

Neuman, Y. (2004). What does pain signify? A hypothesis concerning pain, the immune system and unconscious pain experience under general anesthesia. *Medical Hypotheses* (online periodical), *63*(6).

Norton, P. J. & Asmundson, G. J. G. (2003). Amending the fear-avoidance model of chronic pain: What is the role of physiological arousal? *The Behavior Therapist, 34*, 17–30.

Otis, J. D., Keane, T. M. & Kerns, R. D. (2003). An examination of the relationship between chronic pain and post-traumatic stess disorder. *Journal of Rehabilitation Research and Development, 40*(5) 397–406.

Ottarsdottir, U. (2018). Processing emotions and memorising coursework through memory drawing. *Art Therapy Online, 9*(1), 1–44.

Powell, L. & Faherty, S. L. (1990). Treating sexually abused latency age girls. *The Arts in Psychotherapy, 17*(1), 35–47.

Rankin, A. (1994). Tree drawings and trauma indicators: a comparison of past research with current findings from the diagnostic drawing series. *Art Therapy, Journal of the American Art Therapy Association, 11*(2), 127–130.

Ray, A. L. & Zbik, A. (2001). Cognitive behavioral therapies and beyond. In: Tollison, C. D., Satherwaite, J. R. & Tollison, J. W. (2001). *Practical Pain Management*, 189–208. Philadelphia, PA: Lippincott, Williams & Wilkins.

Read, J. P., Stern, A. L., Wolfe, J. & Ouimette, P. C. (1997). Use of a screening instrument in women's health care: detecting relationships among victimization history, psychological distress, and medical complaints. *Women & Health, 25*(3), 1–3.

Rhinehart, L. & Engelhorn, P. (1982). Pre-image considerations as a therapeutic process. *The Arts in Psychotherapy, 9*, 55–63.

Rhinehart, L. & Engelhorn, P. (1984). The full rainbow-Symbol of individuation. *The Arts in Psychotherapy, 11*, 37–43.

Rhyne, J. (1973). *The Gestalt Art Experience.* Pacific Grove, CA: Brooks/Cole.

Rinfret, M. (2000). Intégration des écoutes psychologiques et somatiques. *Revue Québécoise de Psychologie, 22*(1) 39–56.

Rothschild, B. (2000). *The Body Remembers. The Psychophysiology of Trauma and Trauma Treatment.* New York, NY: W. W. Norton & Company.

Russell, J. (1995). Art therapy on a hospital burn unit: A step towards healing and recovery. *Art Therapy, Journal of the American Art Therapy Association, 12*(1), 39–45.

Salois, P. G. (1995). Spiritual healing and PTSD. *NCP Clinical Quarterly* (online periodical), *5*(1).

Scaer, R. C. (2001). *The Body Bears the Burden. Trauma, Dissociation, and Disease.* Binghamton, NY: The Haworth Medical Press.

Schnurr, P. P. (1996). Trauma, PTSD, and Physical Health. *The National Center for Post-Traumatic Stress Disorder Research Quarterly, 7*(3).

Schnurr, P. P. S. III, Spiro, A. & Paris, A. H. (2000). Physician-diagnosed medical disorders in relation to PTSD symptoms in older male military veterans. *Health Psychology, 9*(1), 91–97.

Schnyder, U. & Cloitre, M. (2015). *Evidence-based Treatments for Trauma-related Psychological Disorders: a Practical Guide for Clinicians.* Cham: Springer.

Schore, A. N. (2018). *La Régulation Affective et la Réparation du Soi.* Montréal, QC: Les Éditions du CIG.

Schreiber, S. & Galai-Gat, T. (1993). Uncontrolled pain following physical injury as the core-trauma in post-traumatic stress disorder. *Pain, 54*(1), 107–110.

Shapiro, F. (2002). EMDR and the role of the clinician in psychotherapy evaluation: towards a more comprehensive integration of science and practice. *Journal of Clinical Psychology, 58*(12), 1453–1463.

Sharp, T. J. & Harvey, A. G. (2001). Chronic pain and post-traumatic stress disorder: Mutual maintenance? *Clin Psychol Rev, 21*, 857–877.

Shepard, R. (1967). Recognition memory for words, sentences, and pictures. *Journal of Verbal Learning and Verbal Behavior, 6*(1), 156–163.

Shipherd, J. C., Beck, J. G., Hamblen, J. L., Lackner, J. M. & Freeman, J. B. (2003). Preliminary Examination of treatment for posttraumatic stress disorder in chronic pain patients: a case study. *Journal of Traumatic Stress, 16*(5), 451–457.

Siegel, B. (1994). *L'Amour, la Médecine et les Miracles.* Paris: J'ai lu.

Solomon, S. (2005). Chronic post-traumatic neck and head pain. *The Journal of Head & Face Pain* (online periodical), *45*(1), 53–67.

Spencer, L. B. (1997). *Heal Abuse and Trauma Through Art: Increasing Self-worth, Healing of initial wounds, and creating a sense of connectivity.* New York, NY: Charles C. Thomas.

Sykes Wylie, M. (2004). The limits of talk; Bessel van der Kolk wants to transform the treatment of trauma. *Psychotherapy Networker, 28*(1).

Taylor, S. & Koch, W. J. (1995). Anxiety disorders due to motor vehicle accidents: Nature and treatment. *Cl Psychol Rev. 15*, 721–738.

Ticen, S. (1990). Feed me…cleanse me…sexual trauma projected in the art of bulimics. *Art Therapy, Journal of the American Art Therapy Association, 7*(1), 17–21.

Tolle, E. (2004). *The Power of Now.* Vancouver, BC: Namaste Publishing.

Turk, D. C. & Winter, F. (2020). *The Pain Survival Guide: How to Become Resilient and Reclaim Your Life.* Washington, DC: American Psychological Association.

Van der Kolk, B. A. (1987). *Psychological Trauma.* Washington, DC: American Psychiatric Press.

Van der Kolk, B. A. (1994). The body keeps the score. *Review of Psychiatry, 1,* 253–265.

Van der Kolk, B. A. (1996). The body keeps the score: approaches to the psychobiology of posttraumatic stress disorder. In: Van der Kolk, B. A., McFarlane, A. C., Weisaeth, L. *Traumatic Stress: the Effects of Overwhelming Experience on Mind, Body, and Society,* 214–241. New York, NY: Guilford Press.

Van der Kolk, B. A. (1998). Neurobiology, Attachment and Trauma. Presentation at the annual meeting of the International Society for Traumatic Stress Studies, Washington, DC.

Verrier, P. (2003). Docteur, ce n'est pas dans ma tête, j'ai vraiment mal. *Le Médecin du Québec, 38*(6), 53–60.

Vlaeyen, J. W. S. & Linton, S. J. (2000). Fear-avoidance and its consequences in musculoskeletal pain: A state of the art. *Pain, 85,* 317–332.

Waller, C. S. (1992). Art therapy with adult female incest survivors. *Art Therapy, 9* (3), 135–138.

Wammes, J. D., Meade, M. E. & Fernandes, M. A. (2016). The drawing effect: Evidence for reliable and robust memory benefits in free recall. *The Quarterly Journal of Experimental Psychology, 69*(9), 1752–1776.

Weil, A. (2014). *Spontaneous Healing: How to Discover and Enhance Your Body's Natural Ability to Maintain and Heal Itself.* Kindle Edition.

Yates, M. & Pawley, K. (1987). Utilizing imagery and the unconscious to explore and resolve the trauma of sexual abuse. *Art Therapy, Journal of the American Art Therapy Association, 4*(1), 27–35.

Zinker, J. (2006). *Le thérapeute en tant qu'artiste. Écrits de 1975 à 2001.* Paris: L'Harmattan.

# Author Index

Asmundson, G. J. G., Wright, K. D., McCreary, D. R. & Pedlar, D. 16, 17
Asmundson, G. J. G., Coons, M. J., Taylor, S. & Katz, J. 16, 17

Brillon, P. 32
Brunet, A., Orr, S. P., Tremblay, J., Robertson, K., Nader, K. & Pitman, R. K. 52

Camic, P. M. 12, 25–26
Carey, L. 27, 47–48
Chapman, L. 15
Chopra, D. 63
Coan, J., Dchaefer, H. & Davidson, R. 73

Duchastel, A. 35, 78, 86, 87

Ecker, B., Ticic, R. & Hulley, L. 51–53, 55, 60, 62

Gantt, L. & Tinnin, L. W. 29
Golub, D. 42
Goswami, A. 63–64, 73, 77
Grant, M. & Threlfo, C. 19

Hamel, J. 53, 56, 64, 67, 70, 74, 123, 126–127, 129, 141
Hass-Cohen, A. & Findlay, J. C. 29, 62
HeartMath Institute 74–75, 77
Hosoi, M. 20
Howard, R. 43–44

Jacobson, M. 26–27, 32–33
Jobin, A.-M. 34, 36, 72–73, 85
Johnson, D. R. 43
Jones, J. G. 28
Jung, C. 45

Lambert, J. & Simard, P. 27, 44
Levine, P. 3, 8, 17–19, 33, 41, 46–47, 67, 141
Lindy, J. D., Green, B. L. & Grace, M. 48
Lipton, B. 64, 73, 77

Melzack, R. M. & Walls, P. D. 12
Mills, J. 37, 153–154
Modell, A. H. 57
Moorjani, A. 73–74, 77
Morgan, C. A. & Johnson, D. R. 42, 44
Muraoka, M., Komiyama, H., Hosoi, M., Mine, K. & Kubo, C. 20

Nader, K., Schafe, G. E. & Ledoux, J. E. 52, 62
Norton, P. J. & Asmundson, G. J. G. 17

Ottarsdottir, U. 52

Rhinehart L. & Engelhorn, P. 7–9, 83–84, 86
Rhyne, J. 7, 42
Rinfret, M. 8, 67
Rothschild, B. 17, 46–48, 142

Scaer, R. C. 3, 18–19, 46, 49–50, 115
Shepard, R. 52
Schore, A. N. 53
Sykes Wylie M. 48

Tolle, E. 66

Van der Kolk, B. A. 3, 8, 28, 46–48, 142–143

Wammes, J. D., Meade, M. E. & Fernandes, M. A. 52

Zinker, J. 70

# Subject Index

abreaction 15, 26–27, 32–33, 41
abuse 32, 41; emotional 129; physical 15–16, 129; power 129; sexual 8, 15–16, 27; substance 11, 75; *see also* child
accident 11, 15, 18, 20, 46, 49, 92, 114–115, 118, 132
acupuncture 120, 125
adhesions 89–92
affect 17, 41, 46–47, 52–53, 142; affect restauration techniques 32, 35
agoraphobia 58
AIDS 27
amnesia 28, 43, 146, 151
amplification 7; of symptoms 55–57
amygdala 42, 47, 49, 65, 142
anesthesia 20, 135
anger 28, 33–35, 44, 68, 70–72, 98–99, 101, 119–120, 129–130, 146, 157; retroflected 70, 72; outbursts of 14; *see also* retroflection
anxiety 10, 47, 59–60, 73; sensitivity 16–18; generalized anxiety disorder 58; performance 59
art media 35; psychological impact of art media 45, 88
art process therapy 1, 7, 9, 83, 86, 88, 115, 118
assertiveness 54, self- 119; assertive 115
avoidance 14–16, 58, 148, 150–151, 152, 153; emotional 52–3, 56; fear- 17; mechanism 18
awareness 19, 51, 56, 66, 70, 78, 103, 105, 148, 150, 153

back pain 11, 99, 101, 114
behavior 8, 17, 20, 29, 34, 41, 46–48, 57–58, 60, 131, 147, 149, 151, 157–158; compulsive 28

body: image 52; memories 26; mind-body integration 48; -schema 69
Bowl of light 37, 153–154
brain 47, 49, 60: intuitive 65; left 30, 42, 47, 142, 157; right brain 9, 30, 41–42, 47, 53, 126, 142; right hemisphere 47, 157; *see also* heart-brain
breathing 35, 97, 112, 140
broca's area 42–43, 47
Buddha: buddhist 127, 141
burn victims 11, 27

cancer 8, 26, 27, 63, 73–74, 77, 99
catastrophic: catastrophizing 16, expectation 18, 20
catharsis 8, 44, 104, 105; cathartic 72, 105
clay 8, 33, 53, 60–61, 112, 136, 153–154
cognition: cognitive 17–18, 20, 28, 43, 53, 60, 72, 91; distortions 30; losses 8; restructuring 18, 20; *see also* cognitive behavioral
cognitive behavioral 12, 15, 18, 25, 32
collage 7, 25–26, 33, 37
collapsing mechanisms 64
collective disasters 28
colour(s), color(s) 7, 34, 36, 41–42, 53–56, 67, 72, 83–86, 89, 91, 96, 108, 109, 112, 124, 156–157; healing color 70, 85, 118, 137
consciousness 1–2, 29, 47, 51, 56, 63–67, 70, 73–74, 77–78, 143; *see also* heart; mind; quantum; subconscious
contact boundary 55
cortex 42, 47, 65
counter-experience 52–54, 60–62
creativity 30; creation 42, 72; creative: arts 25–27, 48, 51; process 54, 56, 62, 66–67, 70, 78

death 14, 20, 99, 121, 141, 145, 148, 150; near- 73–74
defense mechanisms 56
de-freezing techniques 32–33
depersonalization 29, 69, 147
depression 10, 17, 34, 69
diagnostic 142; criteria 147, 150; PTSD 15, 46, 145
dialogue techniques 29, 34, 84, 87, 94
disease 1–2, 9–10, 27, 63–64, 74, 77–78, 85, 109, 143
dissociation 15, 19, 26, 36, 46–47, 49–50, 150; dissociative processes 46; *see also* DID; symptom
DID: dissociative identity disorder 27
distress 10, 14–15, 35,132, 146–149, 151–152, 155; emotional 16, 19–20, 42
dreams 28, 121, 145–148, 151; *see also* nightmares
dyspareunia: acquired dyspareunia 9, 120

EMDR (Eye Movement Desensitization and Reprocessing )15, 18–20
emotion(s) 2, 15, 33–35, 41–42, 44, 49, 52–53; 58, 63, 69, 72, 75, 78, 85, 87–88, 118, 121–122, 127, 129, 143, 1478, 149, 151, 157; expression 28, 47, 157; -focused therapy 51; unconscious 118; *see also* avoidance
emotional: side of pain 20; memory reconsolidation: *see* memory
energy 34, 66, 72–73, 75, 114; non–discharged 46; traumatic 19; waves 72; energetic: design 2; dimension 63; sensitivity 75
experiential 52, 66; dissonance 60, 62; journey 101; method 67–68, 70, 78; process 73–74, 108, 110, 112
exposure: -based therapy 18; to interoceptive sensations 18; *in vivo* 15; to traumas, 142, 145–146, 148, 150, 152; *see also* violence

fatigue 17, 86, 109; chronic 9; *see also* symptom
fear(s) 16–17, 34, 47, 51, 53, 56, 58, 67, 73, 146, 149; fear-avoidance model 17
feeling(s) 8, 14, 16, 19, 28–30, 33–34, 37, 44, 48, 50, 54, 84–85, 146–147, 150–151; *see also* felt sense
felt sense 8, 19, 56, 66, 67, 72; heart- 73
fibromyalgia 9, 11, 16

fight-or-flight 29, 51
flashbacks 17; behavioral 48
form(s) 43, 46, 63–64, 85, 121, 156–157
Four Noble Truths 127, 141
four-quadrants method 3, 54, 56, 60, 62, 83, 88, 127, 155
freeze response 19, 29, 49; frozen: in time 46; motor reaction 15; movements 105; part of self 29

gate control theory 12
Gestalt 7, 9, 51, 54; art therapy 56
GRP (Graphic Narrative Processing) 29
grief 28, 95, 157
guilt 15, 28, 61, 65, 121, 146, 149, 151

healing 2, 4, 36, 37, 60, 62, 63–66, 69, 74, 77, 127, 143, 157; color 67, 70, 71–72; "hands-on" 67, 83; metaphor 123, 133, 141; self-healing 65, 67, 73, 78
headaches 11, 54, 118, 120
heart 34–35, 72; -brain 1, 3, 65– 67, 70, 73–75, 77–78; coherence 3, 63, 67–68, 73–74, 78; rate 17; soma 69–71
Humanist: art therapy 7; psychology 9; humanistic approach 7, 32
hypervigilance 42, 66, 147, 152
hypnosis 18, 20, 43
hypothalamus 47, 65

identity 15, 114; reconstruction techniques of 32, 36; *see also* DID
image(s) 3, 17, 41, 44, 46–47, 54, 56–57, 59–60, 62, 67, 83–86, 88, 127, 142, 156–157; self-image 30, 59; *see also* body
imaginary 19, 60, 97, 133
imagination 94, 133, 141
integrity 15, 44, 114; personal integrity restauration techniques 32, 37
intelligence: intuitive 66, 70, 74–75; non-local intelligence 77; of the source design 64, 74
intuition 42, 74; non–local 75, 77; *see also* intelligence; brain
intrusive: distressing memories 145, 148, 150, 152; re-experiencing 45; *see also* symptoms
isomorphism 41–43, 45
ITR (Instinctual Trauma Response) 29

kindling process 49

limbic system 20, 43, 157

meditation 25, 69, 72, 129, 156; with a
  healing color 85
medium 7, 33, 43, 44, 45, 84, 85
memory 15, 43–44, 47, 51–53, 60,
  65, 87; emotional memory reconsolidation 3, 51–52, 60–62, 142;
  procedural 19, 42, 49–50, 114–115,
  118; reconsolidation 29–30, 52–53;
  somatic 9, 30, 46–48; traumatic 26,
  49, 52
metaphor 3, 57, 60; healing 123, 133
mind 47–48, 53, 63–64, 65–67, 78, 127;
  conscious 56, 66, 121; no–mind
  gap 66
motor vehicle accident 11, 18, 49,
  114, 118
movement(s) 7, 19, 41–42, 56; *see also*
  EMDR
MPD (Multiple Personality Disorder)
  26, 27, 32
music 25, 27, 36, 48
muscles: see myofascial pain
mutual maintenance model 17

nervous system 46, 47, 49, 65, 75, 148;
  neurobiological loops 49; neurovegetative overactivation 49; *see also*
  neuro-cardiology, neuroscience
neuro–cardiology 65–66, 74
neuroscience(s) 3, 29, 42, 51, 126,
  155, 158
nightmares 32, 42–44; recurrent,
  recurring 14, 45
nociception: 20

pain(s) 20, 34–35, 51, 54, 62–66, 73;
  acute 1, 10, 26, 83, 86; back 114;
  chronic pain 25, 26, 27, 32, 41,
  45, 46, 83–85, 88, 89–92, 93–96,
  98–103, 107–109, 112–113, 114–119;
  emotional aspects of 20; myofascial
  pain 49–50; phantom limb 20; *see
  also* dyspareunia; nociception;
  whiplash
posture 49–50, 106; asymmetrical
  postural patterns 49–50
presence 66, 70, 72, 77–78; heightened
  state of presence 74
proprioception 29; proprioceptive:
  manifestations 8; process 122
protocols: art therapy protocols for
  PTSD treatment 25, 29–30

psychotherapy 12, 53–54, 62, 114, 118,
  121; art psychotherapy 62, 120
PTSD (Post-Traumatic Stress Disorder)
  2–3, 11, 14–15, 16–20, 25, 27–29, 32,
  37, 41–42, 44–46, 49, 142–143, 145;
  *see also* trauma; memory; protocols;
  symptoms

Quantum 67, 73–74; healing 2, 63–64;
  leap in consciousness 77–78; model
  3, 63–65, 143; physics 2, 63, 77;
  *see* also self

reconsolidation 3, 29–30, 51–54, 60, 62;
  reconsolidation therapy 52; *see also*
  memory
recovery 56, 133; spontaneous 77
retroflection 34, 68, 130; retroflected
  anger 34, 70, 72

safe haven 15, 32, 36; safe place 19,
  28, 58
sandplay therapy 26–28, 33, 48
scribble 94, 110, 130
SE (Somatic Experiencing Approach)
  8, 18–19
self 2, 29, 34, 42, 49, 54, 57, 60, 61,
  64, 69–70, 75–76, 100–101, 105,
  130–131, 147, 150, 154, 157;
  -efficacy 18, 48; -esteem 28, 37,
  153; fragmented 72; healing 65, 67,
  78; image 30, 44, 59; -love 72–74;
  -mutilating 68; -portrait 30, 35;
  Quantum Self 73; -reliant 131;
  *see also* freeze
sensation 8–9, 17, 18–19, 34, 35, 41,
  46–48, 49–50, 53–55, 59, 69, 72,
  83–87, 155–156; interoceptive
  18, 122
sexuality 54, 121; *see also* abuse,
  violence
shared vulnerability hypothesis 17
shock 92, 115
SIBAM model 17, 41–42, 46–47, 142
silhouette 68, 83, 85–86, 116,123–126,
  132–134
sleep 14, 45, 147, 149, 151
somatic: coherence 2, 72, 74; dissociation 46, 49; re-experiencing 17;
  *see also* heart soma; memory; SE,
  symptom
somatization 16, 49
source design 64, 67, 73–75, 77–78
startle response 14, 29, 45, 147, 152

"stepping in" technique 26, 33
stress 28, 47; acute stress disorder 15, 150; reduction and relaxation techniques 32, 36; see also PTSD
subconscious 47, 101
symptom(s) 20, 48, 52–55, 60–62, 64, 66; amplification 56–58; avoidance 151; deprivation 55, 58–59; dissociative 46–47, 147, 149–151; fatigue 60–61; PTSD 14–18; 32, 37, 42, 49; re-experiencing 16, 42; somatic 28, 49, 54; urinary urgency 48; *see also* intrusion; whiplash

*temenos* 9, 44, 78, 108
transformation 51, 70, 72–73, 105, 127; process 101

trauma 2, 14–20, 27–30, 41–42, 46–52, 109, 114, 137, 141–143, 146, 151–152; memories 15, 27–28, 47, 142; medical trauma 26; treatment 32–33, 36, 47; *see also* abuse, protocols

veterans 11, 16, 27, 42, 44
vibration(al): energy 75; frequency 63, 66; matter 63–64; space of infinite love 73
violence: exposure to 14–15; sexual 145, 148, 150
visualization 36, 86

whiplash: symptoms 11, 49, 114, 118
wound 34, 137; burnt 132

For Product Safety Concerns and Information please contact our EU
representative GPSR@taylorandfrancis.com Taylor & Francis Verlag GmbH,
Kaufingerstraße 24, 80331 München, Germany

Printed and bound by CPI Group (UK) Ltd, Croydon, CR0 4YY

01/05/2025

01858508-0001